W9-AZW-568

Immune for Life

Also by Arnold Fox, M.D. and Barry Fox, M.F.A.

DLPA to End Chronic Pain and Depression
The Beverly Hills Medical Diet
Wake Up! You're Alive

How to Order:

Quantity discounts are available from the publisher, Prima
Publishing & Communications, P.O. Box 1260IL, Rocklin,
CA 95677; telephone (916) 624-5718. On your letterhead include information concerning the intended use of the books
and the number of books you wish to purchase.

U.S. Bookstores and Libraries: Please submit all orders to St.
Martin's Press, 175 Fifth Avenue, New York, NY 10010;
telephone (212) 674-5151.

Immune for Life

Live Longer and Better by
Strengthening Your "Doctor Within"

Arnold Fox, M.D.
Barry Fox, M.F.A.

Prima Publishing & Communications
P.O. Box 1260IL
Rocklin, CA 95677
(916) 624-5718

Production by Robin Lockwood, Bookman Productions
Typography by Col D'var Graphics
Jacket design by The Dunlavey Studio

Prima Publishing & Communications
Rocklin, CA

Library of Congress Cataloging-in-Publication Data

Fox, Arnold, 1928–
  Immune for life.

  Bibliography p.
  Includes index.
  1. Health.   2. Holistic medicine   3. Immunity.
  I. Fox, Barry.   II. Title.
  RA776.5.F69   1989   613   88-32480
  ISBN 0-914629-80-8

89 90 91 92 RRD 10 9 8 7 6 5 4 3 2 1

Printed in the United States of America

Dedicated to Eleanor, Moishe, and Phil.
The world was a better place because you were here.

Our "Doctor Within"

Most of the diseases we get are really failures of our "doctor within." You can call them heart disease, or infections, or herpes, or stroke, or high blood pressure, or cancer, or AIDS, or the common cold, but the truth is that they are all due to a breakdown in our natural defenses. If your immune system is strong, you can shrug off most diseases. That's where the Immune for Life program can help you . . . possibly save you.

Whatever shape you're in, you can begin to make changes in your habits and lifestyles to stop harming your "doctor within" and commit yourself to a proven program of Super Foods, energizing vitamins and minerals, sensible moderate exercise, positive affirmations, visualizations and meditative relaxation that will put you on the road to glowing, vibrant health and happiness.

Starting right now—*today*.

CAUTION: It's always a good idea to seek the advice of your physician before beginning or changing to a new diet, supplement or exercise program. If you have any medical condition, or are on prescription or non-prescription medications, see your physician before altering or discontinuing their use, and certainly before embarking on the Immune for Life program. In any case, I advise you to discuss all aspects of the Immune for Life program with your doctor. He or she may wish to tailor the program to your specific needs.

Acknowledgments

I've delivered many babies in my time. It was not simply a pleasure, it was akin to the ineffable joy that one gets in the presence of the higher power. When the head emerges from the birth canal even the most veteran doctor is excited. Next come the shoulders, then the rest of the body.

What is a baby? A bundle of potential with the ability to change the world, to do good, to be an Albert Schweitzer, to bring world peace, to end hunger. A bundle of potential. A book too, is a bundle of potential. With the birth of a new book the authors watch for signs that their endeavor is fulfilling its potential. So many people helped give birth to this book. Our editor, Murray Fisher, guided us from the early days, giving our writing shape and substance. Ben Dominitz, the publisher, had the vision to see what might be. Our agents, Jim and Rosalie Heacock, advised us in selecting the topic and writing the early chapters.

Norman Vincent Peale has referred to my coauthor and son, Barry, and I as "an amazing father and son team." But our work is more than the product of two people: The whole family is involved. Luckily, the Foxes are used to working together. For years the whole family entertained at hospitals, senior citizens homes, convalescent homes, parties, and even political campaigns. But that's a whole book in itself, which Barry and I will write later. The foremost ingredient for our family recipe is Hannah, wife and mother, the guiding light and strong center of family love, always there with ideas and help.

Barbara and her husband Danny keep us looking for the newness of life, the extra something that turns the ordinary into the extraordinary. Barbara is always there to help, and whatever she does, it's with a big smile.

My oldest son, Howard, and his wife of ten years, Robin, are a loving couple with three children: Melanie, age 7; Josh, age 5; and little Andrew, who just turned two. The joy this branch of the Fox family gets from life is inspiring and infectious. Being with them makes us happier, and because happier, healthier.

Steven, our brand new attorney, is spending this year working with a federal judge in Tennessee, learning the ins and outs of the law firsthand. Letters go back and forth between here and Tennessee. He sends me something to read, and I send him something back. Always, we send much love written between the lines.

Eric, my son the doctor, is in New York with his wife Fienie, completing his residency in Anesthesia. He and Fienie bring a lot of sincerity and warmth to the family—and he always makes me laugh. I'm so glad that medicine is going to get such a wonderful and knowledgeable M.D. It's only thirty years ago that I was a resident— it seems like I only blinked my eyes, and now he's there, teaching me the latest. That's the way life is.

Bruce always keeps us learning. The youngest of the Foxes, his approach to life spurs me to constantly examine my own values. He keeps us in touch with the teenager's view of life, which may be the view of the future.

This is the fourth book that Barry and I have written and published. We've worked through the books, from conception to birth, and now we wait to see if the potential and promise will be fulfilled. You know, it wasn't so long ago that I waited and watched Barry emerge into this world. And now, with fatherly pride, I observe my son and fellow author. I've seen him live up to his potential, and even more!

Now we both sit back and wait and watch, thanking God and all those who helped us deliver *Immune for Life* to you.

I've wanted to be a doctor since I was 12. I'm tickled pink that I, a boy from South Philly became a country doctor teaching health and happiness here in Beverly Hills, California. I pinch myself every day to see if it's real.

Contents

The Immune for Life Program

Chapter 1

Dr. Fox's Immune for Life Program

I once knew a strong, healthy grandmother, 72 years young, who lived an active life, driving her friends to club meetings and to the store, working part time, running errands for her sickly neighbors. One day she told me she had had a cold for three weeks; it simply wouldn't go away. When it persisted, I insisted she be thoroughly checked out. The diagnosis was grim: leukemia, a cancer of the white blood cells.

I visited her in the hospital every day, horrified at the rapid progress of the disease. This once-vibrant woman lay in bed, too weak to move, mouth agape, eyes dull. Shortly before she died she said to me, "I was so healthy. Why did I get sick?" Unable to answer her question, I turned away, tears in my eyes. I had no answers for her. Neither could I offer any help. It was especially painful because this woman was my mother.

Like many people of her generation, she never thought about health or illness. Health was something you took for granted— until you lost it. Today we have a different approach, taught to us by painful experience. We're learning that health is a treasure to be guarded, a single, precious flower to nurture and protect. The good gardener is rewarded with a wonderful harvest of health and happiness.

Ironically, we can thank disease for forcing us to focus our attention on health. In my 28 years of practicing medicine I've seen scares come and go. Fears of tuberculosis and polio were replaced by fright over heart disease and cancer. A new scourge, herpes, came into the picture in the early 1980s. Herpes hysteria had hardly settled down before it was nearly swept aside by the panic over AIDS (acquired immune-deficiency syndrome) and other immune-system diseases. New diseases seem to be popping out of thin air. Some of them we learn to cure. Others we haven't—not yet, anyway.

The patients who come to my office every day are frightened. "What's going to get me?" they wonder. A heart attack? Cancer? A stroke? Diabetes? Will I be crippled by arthritis or made helpless by Alzheimer's disease? Will I wind up in a hospital or a rest home, unable to care for myself?

Recently, a very attractive 39-year-old businesswoman, the sales director for a national cosmetic company, sat in my office nervously rubbing one hand against the other. The divorced parent of a ten-year-old boy, she travels extensively on business.

"You know what it's like, Dr. Fox," she said. "You get to a city, you're running around all day; at night you go to your hotel, and you're lonely. So you've got a 'boyfriend' you see 10, 12 times a year, or maybe you meet someone at a hotel. I don't jump into bed with any guy, but I'm not married and I get lonely on the road. But not any more. I've been getting away from that in the past six months. I'm so scared of getting sick, of catching something that will wreck my immune system. I don't care how lonely I get, I'm not doing it anymore. Not until they figure out a way to protect you from all those diseases you can catch. Not just AIDS, but all of them."

Many Diseases with One Target: Your Health

"Big" diseases such as AIDS are grabbing the headlines. But as a physician, an Internist and a Cardiologist, I can tell you that the diseases you read about, terrible though they may be, are only the tip of the iceberg. The number-one killer in this country is heart disease: 50 percent of us will fall prey to heart conditions. Cancer will claim another 20 percent. About 36 million of us are suffering from arthritis; another 10 million have diabetes, which is the leading cause of new cases of blindness, about five thousand per year. An additional 20 thousand people a year have toes, feet or legs amputated because of diabetes. Add to that the innumerable colds and flus, the general aches and pains, the fatigue and weariness, the listleness and unhappiness I see so much of.

Martha R. is a 42-year-old mother of three who came to my office and announced, "I haven't been healthy in ten years. They ought to make a TV show about me, 'What's My Disease?' On the average I have four colds a year, the flu twice, six to eight asthma attacks, migraines twice a month. I have to drag myself out of bed every morning, my life is boring and nothing makes me laugh. Oh, and my last doctor said I also have hypoglycemia."

Diagnosis: Poor Health Across the Country

If you think you have nothing to worry about because your doctor has told you you're in average health, think again:

- The average American in average health has the average heart attack.
- The average American in average health gets the average cancer, diabetes, stroke.
- The average American is tired and unhappy.
- The average American has no idea what it's like to feel really great.

- The average American stumbles from doctor to doctor, pill to pill, disease to disease—until he dies.
- The average American dies too young, feeling old and worn out.
- The average American is scared—and should be!

As a physician who has worked on the front lines of crisis medicine, treating patient after patient in the intensive care units and coronary care units, and seeing thousands more in my office, I can tell you that the average American is a medical disaster waiting to happen.

One of my patients complained: "It started about a year ago, Dr. Fox. I had a cold, and then a flu, then another cold, then another flu, and my nose was always running and one thing after another. No matter what I did, I couldn't get well. A whole year of being sick! What's wrong with me?"

What was wrong? For any number of reasons, his body's defenses were down. As you will learn, colds, flus and other problems are clues, telling us to take a look at the patients' entire defense system. The colds and flus aren't diseases in themselves; they are symptoms of the underlying problem, which is a breakdown of the "doctor within."

Your "Doctor Within": The Key to Health and Happiness

Despite the self-imposed odds against our doing so, we manage to struggle along, living in fair or poor health into our 60's and 70's; some of us to our 80's and 90's. That we do live—and sometimes flourish—for so long is a tribute to our "internal physician."

Your "doctor within" is an amazing collection of cells, proteins, glands and organs inside your body, genetically programmed to keep you vibrantly healthy and happy. In a sense, the "doctor within" you is you. The heart that pumps fresh blood to all the billions of cells in your body is part of your "doctor within." So are the kidneys that filter out waste products; the endorphin hormones that block certain pain signals and lift your mood; the white blood cells that attack invading germs. Everything in your body that contributes to and fights for your health, happiness and longevity is part of your "doctor within."

The Immune System: Your Built-in Department of Defense

The immune system is one of the major components of your "doctor within." To be immune is to be protected, to have resistance, to be exempt. That's what your immune system is designed to do—protect you and give you resistance against disease. Your immune system is responsible for fighting off bacteria, viruses, fungi, cancer cells and other antigens (things which challenge the immune system). It's genetically programmed to swing into action as soon as disease rears its ugly head.

Germs are all around us, on us and in us. They're on our clothes, in our food, in the air we breathe. If all it took to make us sick was for a germ to land on us, we'd all have died years ago. But we live, we thrive, because that part of our "doctor within" called the immune system maintains a constant vigil inside our body, always ready to destroy diseases before they harm us.

There are many parts to your immune system. You may have heard these names: T-cells, B-cells, phagocytes, complements, interferon, antibodies, interleukin. These are just some of the "immune warriors" your "doctor within" uses to fight disease. You can spend years studying the many fascinating details of the immune system, and I'll tell you more about it in Part Three (page 269). But for now, the important thing to remember is that there is a powerful disease-fighting system within your body.

Many years ago, as a resident in Internal Medicine at Los Angeles County Hospital, I was in charge of the adult infectious-disease ward. For 10 to 15 hours a day I was exposed to just about every infectious illness you can imagine. These patients had tuberculosis, meningitis, the very deadly septicemia and other dangerous diseases. They coughed and sneezed on me; I got their blood, sweat and even feces on my hands. But I didn't "catch" any of their diseases. My "doctor within" kept me in perfect health.

Some time later, I was rotated out of the infectious-disease ward and into surgery. Months later I came down with meningitis, a potentially deadly infection of the covering of the brain. Why? None of the people I was treating had meningitis. I wasn't near anyone with meningitis who could have "given" me the disease. What happened was that I was working double shifts, going to every class and lecture offered and moonlighting besides. In other words, I ran my immune system into the ground. Without immune-system protection I was "easy pickings" for any disease. If not meningitis, I would have "caught" something else.

Colds, flus, polio, herpes, cancer, forms of arthritis and other disorders are all symptoms of immune-system dysfunction. AIDS is the immune system disorder getting the most press at the moment, but terrible as it is, it's far from being the only immune-system disease. When I check the blood of patients who "just don't feel good" I may find EB (Epstein-Barr) virus, a member of the herpes virus group that causes infectious mononucleosis and other problems. Or I may find a virus such as CMV (cytomegalic virus), which can cause an immune-system disorder that may leave you feeling terrible, with enlarged glands and a sore throat. A sore throat may not bother you too much, but remember that CMV is attacking and weakening your immune system. With your immune system "on the run" you're more susceptible to other diseases.

Under ideal conditions your immune system would keep you free from many diseases, from colds to cancer. Unfortunately, we don't live in an ideal world. Your goal, therefore, is to use the Immune for Life program to make your immune system as strong as it can possibly be. Remember: the stronger your immune system, the better your health.

Not too long ago I evaluated a 45-year-old magazine editor who was losing weight. At first he had thought it was fine: "I'm overweight anyway." But the weight loss became associated with a rumbling in the abdomen and, later, loose stools. He soon experienced pain in the bones of his extremities. To top off his problem, the mild cough he had had for weeks became more severe.

"I finally realized I was walking like an old man!" he said. "What's wrong with me?" The examination and various tests quickly revealed that his immune system was shot. He was suffering from pneumocystis carinii—an opportunistic infection associated with AIDS—and had other medical problems as well. The AIDS virus severely weakened his immune system, allowing other diseases to strike. This man is now receiving chemotherapy treatment, but the outlook is poor.

I once treated a 36-year-old woman who was complaining of frequent episodes of loose, watery stools, often accompanied by lower abdominal pains. "It's been going on for a month now, Dr. Fox. What is it?" she asked.

Examination of her stool revealed a parasite called *Giardai lamblia*. The same parasite had been detected years ago in a routine examination conducted by her previous physician. Because the parasite was being kept under control by her immune system and wasn't causing any trouble, the doctor had decided that treatment wasn't necessary. But then stress and poor diet caused her immune system to falter. It could no longer control the parasite, and her troubles began.

A Cold, or Cancer?

Which signs and symptoms suggest immune system malfunction? They are varied and often very subtle. Fatigue, cough, malaise, fever, insomnia, skin problems, muscle wasting, muscle pain, unusual hair loss, eye problems, stomach problems, loss of taste, bleeding gums, enlargement of the neck glands, urinary-tract infections, pains and swelling of the legs and feet, bone pains, numbness and tingling of the extremities and difficulty in walking can all point to immune problems. So can depression, irritability, the blues, difficulty staying asleep, inability to concentrate, disorientation, dementia and other disorders.

The point is that various problems, which often seem minor in themselves, can signal any number of immune-system disorders, from a cold to cancer. For a closer look at signs and symptoms of some specific immune-system diseases, see page 283.

Your Mind: The Immune System's Partner in Your Health

The immune system, however, is only one part of your "doctor within." And the immune-system diseases, scary as they are, are only one type of disorder that may strike us. Millions of Americans are suffering from depression, unhappiness, anxiety, irritability and other emotional problems. Research is proving what we've suspected for years—that the thoughts you think have a profound impact on your physical health. And many of us have minds filled with the kind of unhappy thoughts that invite disease.

Recent studies have demonstrated the existence of physical and chemical links between the mind and the immune system. That connection, and the effect one has on the other, is sometimes called psychoneuroimmunology. "Psycho" and "neuro" refer to the brain and nervous system, "immuno" refers to the immune system.

Don't worry about the ten-dollar words. The key point is that the brain greatly influences the levels of various chemicals throughout your body. Not enough of some chemicals, or too much of others, can incite all kinds of problems, including depression, heart attacks and even cancer. Your thoughts change your biochemistry, and your biochemistry affects your health and happiness. So it behooves us to keep our thoughts as happy and positive as we possibly can.

"I was fired last week," said the young woman slumped in a chair. "My ad agency job depended on my making enthusiastic presentations of my ideas. I believe I have the talent, everyone says I do, but I just can't seem to get going. I can't get excited about anything anymore. I used to, all the time. In fact, people thought I was hyper. Now I'm like a blob; I just sit there all day. And I've been feeling sick for months. One thing after another."

This woman was caught up in the cycle of depression, disease, more depression, more disease. Being unhappy made her sick; being sick made her unhappy. And each round left her sicker and more depressed. My examination and blood tests revealed that her immune system was off balance. Luckily she was able to implement my recommendations and lick the problem.

Thinking Yourself Sick

At age 25, John was sitting on top of the world; at least, he should have been. The scion of a wealthy and distinguished family, he was bright, well educated, well built and handsome, with a wry wit that people loved. He was also listless, uninterested in others or himself— and suffered from severe ulcerative colitis.

By the time I saw him, he had had the colitis for two years. Every day he had several watery, often bloody stools. His weight had dropped from a muscular 165 to a gaunt 135 pounds. Switching to the higher-fiber Super Food diet, which I'll describe in Chapter Two, helped control his problem, and he gained back ten pounds. I also insisted that he play racquetball for one hour every day. That helped too. Why racquetball? He mentioned that he had played back in college and enjoyed the friendly competition. More than anything else, I felt, he needed something to spark his interest in life, something to look forward to. If racquetball worked for him, then racquetball it would be.

All went well for six months. His colitis continued

to improve, he gained ten more pounds and he smiled a lot more. Then he stopped playing, and soon the colitis symptoms returned. This time he went to a gastroenterologist who put him on sulfasalazine (the most commonly used drug for inflammatory bowel disease) and cortisone. He became allergic to the sulfasalazine and developed a toxic hepatitis. (This is not too common an occurrence, but it did happen to him.) The cortisone caused him to swell up all over and develop what we call Cushingoid features. Diabetes then occurred as a result.

Now, with these side effects to go along with his colitis, he was really depressed. "There's no mind-body connection, Dr. Fox" he insisted. "I was just born to be unhappy and sick." Try as I might, I couldn't convince him that his unhappy thoughts were largely responsible for his physical ailments.

This young man was unknowingly using the power of his mind to suppress his "doctor within." The negative thoughts that filled his head disrupted his body chemistry. In his case, the result was ulcerative colitis, although it could have been any number of diseases, including cancer.

Stressing Your "Doctor Within"

There's more to stress than being yelled at by your boss or being stuck in traffic. Stress occurs any time your body is called upon to adapt to different circumstances, and there are "good" and "bad" stresses. Anger, negative thoughts and depression are stressors that harm your "doctor within." I'll talk more about stress later, but for now let me say that stress is a major health problem.

Stress contributes to disease. And disease, in turn, is a very stressful event. You must protect your "doctor within" by learning how to avoid the dangerous stress-disease, more-stress-more-disease cycle.

Mr. Grossbaum was an angry 60-year-old man. "That lousy partner of mine!" he used to say, shaking his fist. Mr. Grossbaum and his partner had founded a successful chain of dry cleaning stores on the West Coast. Two excitable men, they never got along. Every time they fought, which was often, Mr. Grossbaum wound up with headaches and stomach pain. Finally, after 25 years of stress, he sold his share of the business to his partner.

He came to see me soon after, complaining of abdominal pain, headaches, high blood pressure, insomnia, nightmares and irritability. "My wife insisted I come," he said. "There's nothing wrong with me that going back and telling off that lousy ex-partner of mine won't cure."

Instead of learning to avoid stress, as I suggested, he called up his old partner to tell him exactly what he thought of him. They yelled at each other on the phone for ten minutes before Mr. Grossbaum ended the conversation by ripping the cord out of the wall and hurling the phone across the room. With his blood pressure sky high, his heart pounding and his hands shaking, he sat down to rest. Five minutes later he had a massive heart attack and died.

Mr. Grossbaum didn't know it, but fighting with his partner—or even thinking about fighting—caused his sympathetic nervous system to spew out high-voltage chemicals that eventually triggered the heart attack.

There's no way to get around it: we've been wired in such a way that our thoughts are felt throughout our bodies. Good thoughts improve our health. Bad, distressful thoughts induce poor health.

We tend to think of our body and mind as distinct entities. It's convenient to separate mind and body for discussion's sake, but they are really both aspects of a singular entity: *you*. What happens in your mind is reflected throughout your body; changing the chemical composition of your cells and body fluids, even affecting your ability to fight off disease. I'll talk more about this in Chapter Five, and show you how to keep your mind filled with the happy, positive thoughts that encourage good health.

Many Names, Many Symptoms: One Disease

Your immune system and your mind are two very important aspects of your "doctor within." Powerful as they are, however, they depend upon all the other components of the "doctor within" to build health and happiness. A weakness in only one part of your "doctor within" is all it takes to encourage disease and/or depression. If the arteries that bring fresh blood to your brain are so clogged that parts of your brain die, or if an injury to your kidneys decreases their ability to filter out wastes, the whole body can suffer grievously.

Your "doctor within" is an interlocking system, so some problems may affect more than one part of your "doctor within." Depression which may be linked to a biochemical imbalance in the brain can trigger the release of high-voltage chemicals that can weaken the immune system. Anger and hatred spur the production of supercharged chemicals which may hasten a heart attack.

Think of your "doctor within" as your shield. If you drop that shield, even a little, you're exposing yourself to disease. What kind of disease? Anything from a heart attack to herpes. But remember, the heart attacks, herpes and other disorders are really symptoms. The real problem is a breakdown of your "doctor within." The weak link may be in the immune system, it may be in the mind, it may be improper regulation of blood pressure or blood sugar. But the immune system, the mind and the mechanisms that oversee blood pressure and blood sugar are all part of your "doctor within."

That's why I say that most of the diseases we get are really failures of our "doctor within." You can call them heart disease or infections or herpes or depression or stroke or high blood pressure or cancer, but the truth is that they are all due to a breakdown of your natural defenses. If your "doctor within" is strong, you can shrug off most diseases. That's what this book is all about: keeping your "doctor within" in tip-top shape.

Assaulting Your "Doctor Within"

"But Arnold" some of my patients say, "If my 'doctor within' is so great, how come I'm always sick? What happened?"

The details and ramifications of the answer are complex, but the answer itself is simple: every day we inflict more and more punishment on our "doctor within." We get in the way. We disrupt the doctor's working conditions. With our diet, our outlook on life and our daily habits, we unknowingly do just about everything we can to stop our "doctor within" from taking care of us.

Disease from the Dinner Plate

You are what you eat, in the sense that food is the raw material with which your body—and your "doctor within"—works. Like any craftsperson, your "doctor within" needs the right tools and materials to do a good job. These include complex carbohydrates, vitamins, minerals, fiber and water. Adequate supplies of protein, plus a small amount of fat, are also necessary.

Most of us eat the Standard American Diet (S.A.D.), which is loaded with fat, protein and simple carbohydrates (sugars), but sadly lacking in complex carbohydrates, fiber, vitamins and minerals. Eating the S.A.D. deprives your "doctor within" of many of the tools needed to build health. At the same time, eating the S.A.D. forces your body to work overtime trying to deal with the mounds of sugar and globs of fat filling your stomach.

Unwrap a stick of butter. Squeeze it in your fist. Rub that butter between your two hands, spread it all over your hands and fingers. That's about as much fat as there is in the food the typical person eats in a day. Feel that fat on your hands. It's thick and gooey. Imagine that much fat in your arteries, turning your bloodstream into a swamp.

As if that weren't enough, the S.A.D., with its large quantities of meat and processed foods, is filled with chemical additives that can hamper—and eventually overcome—your "doctor within." Despite the claims of the food industry, the additives we consume have not been properly tested. Many, in fact, have never really been tested at all: "Grandfather" clauses in the law exempted them from the more stringent requirements. Furthermore, we don't know what happens when the chemicals get together inside your body. Chemical A in your ice cream may be relatively harmless by itself. So might Chemical B in your fast-food French fries. But what happens when the two chemicals meet in your bloodstream or liver? Do they ignore each other? Do they combine? Does A convert B into a more dangerous form? We don't always know what happens. The untold numbers of combinations that can result from eating additive-laden foods have not been studied.

The S.A.D. contributes directly to much of the heart disease we suffer, as well as to strokes, diabetes, arthritis and even cancer. And to the extent that the fatty, sugary, nutrient-poor S.A.D. disrupts your "doctor within" it contributes indirectly to many other problems. To be blunt, the S.A.D. is a killer. And its one and only target is you.

I had known Joan for many years, since my days at Los Angeles County Hospital. Even back then she had a great love for food. She ate juicy hamburgers, steak sandwiches dripping with fat, milk shakes, sausage-and-mustard sandwiches, corned-beef sandwiches and pie for dessert. As we grew older, her weight grew. Although she was never grotesquely fat, there was almost twice as much of her as there should have been. "More of me to love," she said with a smile.

Joan was a friend, not a patient. Still, I tried to warn her of the danger of her diet. "I know what I'm eating isn't good for me," she said. "I've read your books and know about fat and heart disease, and about how fat causes cancers. But I love good food."

When Joan was 45, she discovered a lump in her breast. It was a cancer many feel is related to rich eating— one of the "cancers of affluence." She went through surgery, chemotherapy and radiation. She suffered terribly before becoming another death statistic linking fat to cancer.

Soon after Joan died, a young man came to see me at my office for treatment of a minor ailment. Like many of my patients, he also became a friend. Bob was the type of guy everyone loves to be with. A hard-working, energetic businessman, he was a never-ending source of jokes and stories. He laughed a lot and he ate a lot. Through him, I became acquainted with many of the restaurants between Beverly Hills and the beach. All the maitre d's and waiters knew him: a big spender, a big tipper and a big eater with an appetite for nothing but the richest foods.

Having recently watched my friend Joan die of cancer, I cautioned Bob: "Go easy on the fat. Too much can cause a heart attack, or perhaps cancer."

"You only go around once, Arn," he'd answer with a hearty laugh.

His "go-around" almost came to an abrupt end one night when he woke up gasping for breath, with an incredibly painful sensation spreading across his chest, up his neck and down his left arm. Luckily, his wife knew CPR (cardiopulmonary resuscitation) and kept him alive until the paramedics arrived.

Having survived the heart attack, Bob was fortunate enough to have a second chance—but not wise enough to take advantage of it. I showed him pictures of arteries clogged by the fat and cholesterol he ate so much of. I described how the fat he consumed made his red blood cells sticky and sluggish. I explained that switching to a low-fat, low-cholesterol diet would add years to his life and life to his years.

But Bob wouldn't change his eating habits. Since the heart attack, he's had two coronary artery bypass surgeries and has developed cancer of the colon. After all that he still stubbornly refuses to give up his rich foods. "You only go around once, Arn," he keeps telling me. True, you do only go around once. But that go-around is meant to be lived. I don't call having a heart attack, two heart surgeries and cancer, living. I call that a slow, painful death.

Poisoning Your "Doctor Within"

Our "doctor within" is also forced to deal with the multitude of environmental pollutants that abound in our chemical world. When I taught a class in Physical Diagnosis to a group of medical students, I used to paraphrase Hippocrates: "When you go to patients' houses, you should ask them what sort of pains they have, what brought them on, how many days they have been ill, are their bowels working and what sort of food do they eat?" Today we have to ask an additional question: What toxins (poisons) are you exposed to in your home and workplace? We live in an environment saturated with man-made chemicals, many of them very dangerous to our health. They're in our food, our air, our water, our homes, our clothes, our cars, our offices.

I see more and more people who are complaining of vague symptoms and recurrent illnesses that can be traced to the chemical poisoning of our immune system. Laboratory test results often show high levels of pesticides, solvents and other toxic chemicals in patients. Lead, mercury, chloroform, DDT, DDE and many other substances have a depressing effect upon the "doctor within." Quite often the symptoms—fatigue, loss of energy, forgetfulness, personality changes, depression—give us only general clues as to the identity of the culprit.

How much is too much? When it comes to chemical poisoning of the body, we just don't know. New chemical compounds are being introduced at a fast and furious pace. If scientists were to start conducting the rigorous safety tests they should have been doing all along, they would probably never catch up with all the new chemicals.

Government and industry claim that there are "safe" levels for various toxins in the body. That idea is patently absurd. Five to 40 years may pass before chemicals and particles you were exposed to at work, home or school are expressed as a disease. To be safe, I say that any are expressed as a disease. To be safe, I say that any amount is too much. Any risk to our "doctor within" is too great.

This much we do know: worldwide chemical pollution of our air, food, water and environment is reflected in the chemical pollution of our bodies. For example, house and industrial painters, who have worked for long periods in confined spaces and inhaled paint fumes, may suffer from a chronic brain syndrome characterized by fatigue, headaches, dizziness, depression, irritability and memory impairment. Being on guard against the obvious toxins isn't enough. Hobbies such as sculpting, welding and painting, for instance, expose us to various toxins. Common household cleaners are potentially toxic. You may be unwittingly exposed to asbestos in school, at your workplace, even in your own home.

I couldn't figure out what was wrong with the attractive 45- year-old woman who came to me complaining of frequent colds, irritability, nervousness and forgetfulness. "And those are only the major problems" she explained. "I also have dizziness, insomnia and sometimes pain in my stomach."

The laboratory studies I ordered showed that her immune system was out of whack, but not in any of the usual ways. She didn't have AIDS, EB virus, CMV or any other standard immune-system diseases.

As is my custom, I reviewed all her old medical records. There was nothing in the many documents that suggested an answer to her current problems. She worked in a defense plant, making parts for a new, top-secret bomber. Perhaps she had inhaled a chemical at the factory?

"No," she said, "there aren't any chemicals where I work. We have good ventilation, too, so even if there were chemicals, I wouldn't breathe in a lot of them."

"Well," I continued, "what exactly do you do at work?"

"I run a big machine that stamps out metal," she explained. "But it's almost entirely run by computer. I

"How do you clean it?" I wanted to know. She told me that she poured fluid out of an unlabeled can onto the machine and, using her bare hands, rubbed the fluid in to get the grease off of the machine. That was the clue I needed. Suspecting there might be a toxic chemical in the cleaning fluid, I ordered a battery of toxicology tests to be run. The laboratory found large amounts of chloroform in her blood, plus trichloroacetic acid and trichloroethanol in her urine. It turned out that the cleaning fluid contained trichloroethylene, a very dangerous but widely used industrial solvent. Exposure to this chemical, along with other chemicals and their break-down products, can depress the immune system and cause mental depression and such abnormalities of the central nervous system as confusion and uncoordination. In animals, this chemical has even caused liver cancer.

Happily, she adopted my Immune for Life program, transferred to a different part of the factory, and got away from the cleaning fluid. Most of her symptoms disappeared, and her immune-system tests returned to normal. As a special precaution, I had her get rid of the cleaning fluids and other chemical concoctions in her home.

Toxic chemicals are everywhere. There's asbestos in our buildings, mercury in the fish we eat, pesticides in our beef and potentially harmful hormones in our chicken. The DDT that was banned long ago is still in our drinking water and meats. Processed foods are full of potentially toxic substances. The air we breathe can be toxic. Even wallpaper contains pesticides. In our society, it's very hard to avoid toxic chemicals and environmental pollutants. That's why we must do everything we can to protect and strengthen our "doctor within."

Your Doctor Versus Your "Doctor Within"

I was describing the "doctor within" and the immune system recently to a friend of mine. He said, "What's the problem, Arnie? If I get sick, I go to my doctor and he'll give me a shot to fix my immune system."

Unfortunately, our medical system is not the answer. You see, we don't have a health-care system in this country, we have a disease-care system. Disease is fussed over. People suffering from obscure and "glamorous" diseases are given the medical red-carpet treatment. Millions of dollars, hundreds of journals and some of the best minds in this country are devoted to disease. Medical students spend most of their time studying rare diseases and practicing crisis medicine, instead of learning to *prevent* disease by protecting the "doctor within." And health? Health gets lost in the shuffle.

Our medical system has been captured by the disease-loving "Band-Aid philosophers" of medicine, who pay homage to such high-tech procedures as coronary artery bypass surgery, chemotherapy, plasma electrophoresis, PTCA (percutaneous transluminal coronary angioplasty), CAT scans and, lately, MRI (Magnetic Resonance Imaging) scans.

These surgeries and machines are exciting: it's high-tech glamour. What doctor wouldn't want to be in an operating room, replacing one heart with another? Isn't the chance to play God more fun than trying to teach people to eat and think properly? Sure it is, but it doesn't work. There is no Band-Aid that can restore good health once it's gone.

Our medical system has been led astray. And so our medical researchers concentrate on building new hearts, not on keeping the old ones strong and healthy. Hospitals are filled with tons of amazing machinery that can do everything but give people back their health. Bigger and better machines, more surgical techniques, artificial organs; it's a wonder that there's any room left for patients in our medical system.

Doctors are paid large fees to perform surgery, office procedures and laboratory tests. They are paid very little for spending time listening to their patients, for carefully going over their medical and personal histories, for teaching them how to change their life-style.

Medical Fallacy #1:
Disease As Either/Or

To make matters worse, thanks to at least three medical fallacies our physicians often harm our "doctor within." One of these fallacies is the idea that health is an either/or situation, with nothing in between.

We physicians tend to see a patient as either healthy or diseased. If the person is sick, treat the disease. If there is no recognizable disease, then there is nothing to treat. It seems so very simple, but it's not.

Health isn't an either/or state. It ranges from the best to the worst of health. Imagine a HEALTH LADDER. If you're standing on the top of the ladder, you have vibrant health. Standing on the lowest rung, you have a serious disease, such as cancer. We don't jump from the top of the ladder to the bottom, or the bottom to the top. Health and disease do not appear out of thin air. We climb up or down, step by step, passing through the various stages of disease and health.

With VIBRANT HEALTH you feel great at any and every age. Not only do you feel physically fit, you're happy as well. Your emotional and spiritual health are excellent.

One rung down is FAIR HEALTH. In this condition you don't feel bad, but you don't feel great either. You're a little tired, and perhaps you have a vaguely dissatisfied feeling about life. Still, you're not sick, so your doctor usually can't help you.

Next comes the SYMPTOMS rung. Symptoms are the problems you begin to notice, such as shortness of breath, fatigue, headaches, backaches and chest pain. Standing on the SYMPTOMS rung, you feel run down and unenthusiastic about life.

A step below symptoms is the SIGNS rung. Signs are the changes in your health and/or body that we doctors can actually measure. Elevated blood pressure, irregular heart rhythms and abnormal blood counts are signs. Now you have something your doctor can treat, often with pills and injections. From the SIGNS rung, it is still possible to scramble back up the HEALTH LADDER.

When you're down to the MEASUREABLE ILL-NESS rung, you have an easily identifiable illness such as colitis, tumors, ulcers or diabetes. Now your physician is excited; he or she can bring out a full arsenal of drugs, surgeries, CAT scans, angiograms, nuclear magnetic resonance scans and dialysis.

SERIOUS ILLNESS is the next rung down the ladder. By now your health is nearly gone, and your life is in danger. Serious illnesses include heart disease, cancer, uncontrolled diabetes, and strokes. These are the kinds of problems the medical system is geared to deal with. But even if a doctor manages to "cure" you, it's a long climb back up the health ladder. But it can be done.

Below the SERIOUS ILLNESS rung is DEATH.

If you view health and disease as an either/or situation, you're operating under a serious misconception.

Where do we stand on the HEALTH LADDER? Well, most of us are in average health. That puts us on the SYMPTOMS or SIGNS rungs, bad places to be.

Medical Fallacy #2: Ignoring the Real Disease

The second medical fallacy is our habit of looking at symptoms and labeling them as diseases. This approach ignores the real disease altogether.

Medical students aren't trained to look beyond the immediate problem. If the patient has a cold, they are taught, deal with the cold. If the patient has cancer, provide the appropriate treatment. What's wrong with this approach? Why wouldn't you want to treat the cold or cancer?

Treating the obvious ailment is a good idea, but it's only the first step. Most diseases, whether colds or cancers, are really symptoms of a deeper problem. If you treat the symptoms and gloss over the underlying crisis, the problem will come back again and again. Sure, we can try to radiate a cancer or remove it surgically. We might even be successful in the attempt. But what's to prevent the cancer from recurring?

We patch people up, running from one problem to the next, until the entire system breaks down. When that happens, all our expensive surgeries and machines aren't worth a hill of beans.

Medical Fallacy #3:
Being "Mugged" by Germs

A patient once said to me, "I don't know why I keep getting colds. I guess a bunch of germs have decided to keep mugging me."

I told this man that a painter cannot paint until the palette has been prepared: Neither can a builder build until the foundation has been laid nor an airplane land until a landing strip has been built. *Disease cannot "strike" until and unless you allow it to.*

Yes, we unknowingly invite disease by handicapping, even destroying, our natural defenses. And we're doing ourselves more and more damage all the time. If we were to reverse this dangerous trend, if we would work instead to bolster our natural defenses, we could practically wipe out heart disease, eliminate much of the cancer striking us down and greatly reduce the incidence of arthritis, strokes, diabetes, colds, flus, depression, fatigue and many other problems that plague us. We could save billions of dollars in medical costs and increase our work productivity. We could add years to our lives and happiness to our years.

But as long as we think of disease as something that "just happens" to us because we're unlucky, or because we get "mugged" by some germs, we will never take the necessary steps to prevent disease by strengthening our natural defenses. Instead, we'll continue the many health-destructive habits that most of us unknowingly practice.

Dancing the Deadly Disease Dance

Thanks to all these medical fallacies, the average American spends the last years of life dancing the horrible "disease dance." What is the disease dance? It's the frantic stumbling from doctor to doctor, disease to disease, pill to pill and surgery to surgery. The disease dance is a frenzied search for names and solutions to our problems. For most of us, it's a horrid dance that goes on and on, ending only when we die.

There is a word, "iatrogenic," to describe diseases caused by doctors. The drugs we prescribe can cause iatrogenic diseases; so can the different regimens we recommend, as well as the procedures and surgeries we perform. Medical journal articles suggest that unnecessary surgery causes thousands of deaths a year, plus an unknown amount of injury and misery. I remember going to the hospitals some years ago and looking at the surgical schedules. Whole families of kids were having T&As (tonsillectomy and adenoidectomies). More than 90 percent of the T&As were unnecessary; in fact, they were downright dangerous, because they removed parts of the children's immune systems (tonsils and adenoids). How many of these kids later suffered from compromised immune function? How many suffered from unnecessary disease? Doctors also used to radiate enlarged thymus glands in children, in order to shrink them. Today we know that the thymus gland is where the T-cells of the immune system receive their programming. How many people are walking around with a shrunken thymus, and reduced immune ability?

There's another fancy word physicians use to disguise doctor- caused diseases: nosocomial infections. Nosocomial infections are hospital-acquired infections, which are very serious because our hospitals can be the breeding grounds for virulent germs that have evolved to resist the latest superantibiotics we use.

It might even be fair to say that some doctors are at their worst when it comes to prescribing drugs. Our pharmacies are filled with drugs, from simple aspirin to immunosuppressants for transplant patients. Drugs are ubiquitous; medicine chests are full of them. Doctors are busy prescribing common and exotic medications for everything from acne and insomnia to high blood pressure and depression. *We doctors act as if we believe that disease is caused by a shortage of prescription drugs in the body.*

We tend to look upon drugs as our saviors. But every drug, even the common aspirin tablet, has side effects. No medicine is absolutely safe—not one. I don't know how many patients I've seen who were suffering more from the side effects of their medicines than they were from the original problem. The benefits and risks of each and every drug must be weighed by both doctor and patient before medications are prescribed and taken.

Pain medications may result in dizziness, nausea, constipation or diarrhea, gastrointestinal bleeding, headaches and depression, among other problems. The narcotic painkillers are addicting. Antidepressants can cause high blood pressure, irregular heart rhythms, stroke, confusion, anxiety, numbness, nausea, dizziness, anorexia and many other problems. Arthritis drugs may lead to nausea, bloody bowel movements, ulcers, depression, chest pain, high blood pressure and other problems.

I treated a patient, a 45-year-old accountant, who had gone to his physician for a routine physical. Finding that his blood pressure was a little high, the doctor put him on a diuretic called hydrochlorothiazide. This is a medication designed to lower blood pressure by getting rid of excess sodium and water in the body. Unfortunately, the medicine also flushed potassium out of the man's body, so his doctor had to give him a second medication to bring the potassium level back up. Oh yes: the diuretic also caused his cholesterol level to rise.

Meanwhile, because the man didn't change his life-style in any way, the original diuretic soon failed, and his blood pressure went back up. Now his doctor had him take a beta-blocking agent as well. This controlled his blood pressure but caused him to develop fatigue, weakness, depression, episodes of vertigo and an inability to perform sexually. These new problems occurred so insidiously that he didn't connect the symptoms with the medication.

When he went back to see his doctor, lab studies showed that the uric acid in his blood was high. The doctor didn't realize that this was also due to the diuretic. Soon, the man was back in his doctor's office with clinical gout and severe pain and swelling of his large right toe. So he was given a new medication, this one to handle the gout. The diuretic also raised his blood sugar, so he was given yet another drug to lower the blood sugar.

By now a year had passed. He still had the high blood pressure, plus gout with gouty arthritis, low potassium, high cholesterol and diabetes. On top of that he was weak, tired, depressed and impotent.

I realized that the medications were as dangerous as the original problem. By carefully discontinuing all the medications and having him adopt the program described in this book, I eventually resolved the man's medical disorders.

A study conducted for the Armed Forces Institute of Pathology indicated that the deaths of 6 to 12 thousand people a year can be blamed on reactions to drugs prescribed by their physicians. Sometimes it's easy to treat patients who come to see me with a strange collection of symptoms. Taking them off their many medications clears up the problems. But sometimes it's not so easy.

Don't look to doctors, drugs and surgeries for your health and happiness. We physicians can help you battle certain diseases. But health is more, much more, than the absence of disease. The glowing, vibrant health you want depends on you making your "doctor within" as strong as possible. That's where the Immune for Life program can help you.

Become Immune for Life

Take care of your "doctor within" and your immune system—starting now. Please don't wait for the trouble signs to appear, because by then it may be too late. The road to lifelong immunity starts right here, right now, with the Immune for Life program.

The Immune for Life program begins by acknowledging the importance of your "doctor within." I designed the program to, first, stop harming the good doctor and, second, to begin strengthening this ally. Whatever your immune status, you can begin—right now—to make the changes in your habits and life-style to stop harming your "doctor within" and put you on the road to vibrant health and happiness. Here are the basics of the Immune for Life program:

1. Do you know if your diet is sabotaging your "doctor within"? Or how many health-destructive negative thoughts pass through your mind every day? Knowledge is power. Find out whether your life-style and daily habits are helping or harming your "doctor within." In the Immune for Life Workbook that starts on page 192, you'll find a series of quizzes that will help you evaluate your daily habits and thoughts. Taking the quizzes will teach you a great deal about yourself and will point to potential trouble spots for your "doctor within."

2. Stop harming your "doctor within" and immune system with the dangerous Standard American Diet. Instead, add years to your life and life to your years by switching to the Super Food diet. Find out which foods are the Super Foods, with extra power to protect you against cancer, heart disease, strokes, diabetes, depression and other diseases.

3. Make sure your "doctor within" is getting all the vitamins and minerals it needs by adopting the Nutri Prevention program of supplements best suited to your needs. Your program may include DLPA (dl-phenylalanine), a natural and safe nutrient that bolsters the immune system, blocks chronic pain and relieves certain types of depression by protecting and enhancing the endorphin hormones.

4. Meld your mind and body into an invincible barrier against depression, negative thinking, physical and emotional disease. Learn how not to be a stress seeker who risks heart disease and other problems by trying to take on the world single-handed. Find out whether you're a stress phobic, with depressed, unhappy thoughts that increase your risk of cancer and other diseases. Learn to make affirmations and visualizations a part of your everyday Immune for Life program.
5. Discover how brisk walking and other simple exercises can strengthen your "doctor within," bolster your immune system and fight depression.
6. Soothe and simultaneously energize your "doctor within" with Meditative Relaxation. This is an excellent way to dispose of the stress, anger and frustration that are so destructive to your health and happiness.

The Immune for Life program is relatively simple. But it all depends on your making, here and now, a firm commitment to zestful health, happiness and longevity.

Antiaging with Immune for Life

According to the Scriptures, "Moses was 120 years. His vision was undimmed, and his natural powers were unabated. And Moses died."

Moses lived young and strong to a very old age. He didn't have a heart attack in his 50's, nor did he suffer a stroke or any of the other problems that afflict and kill us so early in life. His supercharged "doctor within" kept him going strong until the end. That's the way it should be for all of us. And that's the way it can be!

In many ways, the Immune for Life program is an antiaging blueprint. It helps delay some of the ravages of aging, such as loss of eyesight and hearing, bent posture, arthritis and other ills associated with growing old. One of the most common causes of blindness is arteriosclerosis, a condition in which the tiny blood vessels feeding the eyes are blocked. And by the age of 50, most Americans have some type of demonstrable hearing loss, due to the clogging of tiny arteries in the ears. Adopting the Immune for Life program will help keep your arteries wide open, thus preventing this type of vision and hearing loss. Depression, arthritis and other signs and symptoms of aging can be slowed or prevented.

The Roman orator Cicero said: "Old age must be resisted and its deficiencies supplied." The Immune for Life program is a big step in the direction of supplying the deficiencies and resisting the ravages of aging.

As far as we know, humans can live to a maximum of 115 or 120 years. The average American, however, lives for only about 70 years, and many of those years are difficult, filled with discomfort, disease, depression and fear. My goal is for us to live not only as long as possible but, even more importantly, as healthy as possible.

Our medical system tells us that it can cure many diseases, and it can. But I say it's better not to get sick in the first place. *Prevention is the real cure!* It's about time the medical establishment realized that there is no better therapy than staying healthy. Don't let yourself get to the point where you need coronary artery bypass surgery, chemotherapy, kidney dialysis and all the rest. Concentrate on strengthening your "doctor within," and health, happiness and longevity can really be yours.

Moses said: "I set before you blessing and curse, life and death. Therefore, choose life." My friends, the choice is yours. Choose life, good health and happiness. Be Immune for Life.

Chapter 2

Super Foods

*B*arely a day passes that I don't read of a new study showing the effect of what we eat on our health. Research is proving that the Standard American Diet (S.A.D.) is dangerous to your "doctor within." I tell my patients, however, that they can turn to an ancient book for a quick lesson in nutrition and health. In the biblical story of Daniel you will find a report of perhaps the first nutritional study ever made. In this story we learn that, although the king instructed his steward to feed Daniel and his three friends rich foods and wine, Daniel insisted on eating only vegetables, grains and water. At the end of ten days, Daniel looked healthier and better nourished than the men who ate the king's diet.

Daniel knew that the fatty, sugary foods set on the royal table were unhealthy. Rather than subject his body to that disease—making diet, he ate nutritious vegetables and grains and drank pure, healthy water. Using the men who ate the king's food as a control group, and himself as the experimental group, he demonstrated the benefits of a nutritious, low-fat diet.

Thousands of years have passed since Daniel's nutrition study, but most of us are still eating the king's rich diet. Our Standard American Diet, like the king's diet, is loaded with fat, cholesterol and sugar, and it is low in complex carbohydrates. The S.A.D. is actually worse than the king's diet, because we've added all kinds of toxic chemicals, plus large amounts of caffeine and salt, to our food. I tell my patients to learn to eat like Daniel ate. For when you dine at the "king's table," you're asking for trouble.

From Your Plate to Your "Doctor Within"

Nature has packed an amazing variety of nutrients into the appealing packages we call food. When you look at an apple, you don't think about the carbohydrates, fat, protein, fiber, calcium, iron, phosphorus, vitamin A, niacin, vitamin C and other nutrients it contains. You see and taste an apple.

As soon as you bite into the apple, however, you begin to "unwrap" the package. Chewing continues the process, which is completed by the enzymes in your mouth, stomach and intestines. Soon, the package is completely unwrapped. No longer an apple, it is now a collection of the nutrients that go into the making of an apple. It's the ingredients, not the apple itself, that are absorbed into your body, and many of these ingredients are a big help to our "doctor within." In other foods, however, the ingredients are a mixed blessing, and some are outright harmful. Let's look at the helpful ones first.

CCs for Energy

Complex carbohydrates, or "CCs" for short, are wonderful immune builders. Imagine a table covered with bowls of steaming hot, whole-wheat pasta dishes, brown rice and other grains, fresh-baked whole-grain breads and rolls, and all kinds of vegetables. There are lots of CCs in these foods.

Carbohydrates come in chains of different lengths. CCs are long chains of sugar tightly bound together. Double or single links comprise the simple carbohydrates. In terms of calories, there is no difference between CCs and simple carbohydrates. But it takes the enzymes in your stomach and intestines more time to break up the long chain CCs. This means that your "doctor within" receives a slow, steady supply of energy to work with. And because CCs are generally found in vegetables, fruits and whole grains, when you eat CCs you're also giving your "doctor within" plenty of vitamins, minerals and fiber.

Vitamins and Minerals

Vitamins and minerals are indispensable tools for your "doctor within," performing innumerable jobs in every cell of your body. They keep your bones and muscles strong, your skin clear and smooth. They also help fight cellular poisons, prevent unnecessary blood clotting, allow your brain to communicate with the rest of your body, heal wounds, fight bacteria and viruses, promote growth, form red blood cells and dispose of body wastes. You name it, vitamins and minerals are involved.

The Protein Myth

Along with CCs, vitamins and minerals, you need protein, but only in small amounts. Too much harms your "doctor within." We've been raised to believe the myth that protein is good for you—the more, the better. After all, it builds muscles, right?

Well, it's true enough that protein is the framework upon which your body is built. It's also necessary for the manufacture of enzymes and hormones, and it can be burned for body energy. Protein is important. But more is not better. If you're eating the S.A.D., you may be getting much too much protein, and that can be dangerous. High-protein diets are associated with increased incidence of cancer in experimental animals. In humans, high levels of protein in the diet have also been linked to calcium loss, which can lead to osteoporosis (bone-thinning) and, therefore, to bone fractures. If your kidneys can't excrete the excess protein, your uric acid level will rise and may trigger gout. Another problem is that the high-protein meats and poultry we eat are full of fat and cholesterol.

Excess Fat Equals Excess Disease

I'm sure you're aware of the link between excess fat and heart disease, excess fat and strokes, excess fat and cancer; in fact, excess fat and all kinds of diseases.

Imagine trying to work in an office filled with thick, gooey fat. It's all over your desk, in your drawers, oozing out of the walls, falling from the ceiling. It's packed so thickly over your telephone receiver that you can't hear what your caller is saying. You can't even write, because your papers are covered. You can barely wade through the gunk piled two feet high in the hallway, and when you open the door to the adjoining office you're buried in an avalanche of glop.

How much constructive work could you accomplish in such an environment? None. You'd spend all your time trying to clean up, to get the junk out of there before it destroys the office, and you along with it. How much health-building work can your "doctor within" do if his workplace—your body—is literally covered with fat? If the fat has clogged up and closed your arteries, your "doctor within" can't even get basic nourishment, let alone try to build good health.

We do need fat in our diet, but only in small amounts. Inside the body, small amounts of fat are useful for storing energy, carrying fat-soluble substances through the watery bloodstream, protecting and insulating us. Fat is like protein in that a little bit is good, but too much is dangerous. Unfortunately, the S.A.D. is absolutely loaded with fat. And fat contributes to, or exacerbates, an amazing number of health problems. The "cancers of affluence"—cancers of the breast, colon and rectum, prostate, pancreas, ovaries and uterus—give gravestone testimony to the deadliness of dietary fat. So, do your "doctor within" a favor: keep your fat intake as low as possible.

Cholesterol: Leave It to Nature

Cholesterol is a "good/bad" item: good because it's essential for life, bad because it's associated with clogged arteries and heart disease.

Here's the general rule I explain to my patients: Your body is very good at making all the cholesterol it needs. You don't have to help it out by eating a lot more. In fact, you really don't have to eat any cholesterol at all.

But eat it we do, in large amounts. Working hand in hand with fat, cholesterol plugs up arteries, especially the tiny arteries that supply the heart muscle and brain. When those arteries close up, we may suffer a heart attack or stroke.

The Pick-Me-Up That Lets You Down

Caffeine is another food item we can do without. Many studies have linked caffeine to irregular heart rhythms, increased blood pressure, heart disease, anxiety, the heartburn of gastritis and esophogitis, peptic ulcers, digestive problems and cancer. Ironically, the caffeine we drink to give us a lift eventually does the opposite. Caffeine gets your heart beating faster and increases your blood sugar. That's what gives you the lift. Your body then reacts to the sudden energy surge by gathering up all the blood sugar it can and stuffing it into your cells. Too much sugar, however, is often gathered up. Now your blood sugar is low; you feel fatigued and want another cup of coffee. For many of my patients, every day is a cruel cycle of fatigue, coffee, brief lift, fatigue, coffee, brief lift, fatigue, and on and on.

That's why I call caffeine the pick-me-up that really lets us down, overstimulating our heart and muscles at the same time. It just makes trouble for our "doctor within."

RCs Are Trouble

Refined carbohydrates (RCs) are other foodstuffs your "doctor within" can do without. Like CCs, RCs are carbohydrate (sugar) chains. RCs are CCs that have been chopped up into short chains, then single units, and stripped of the vitamins and minerals associated with CCs. All that's left is the sugar.

You'll find RCs in breads and pastas made from white (processed) flour, in cakes and pies, in sugar, honey, molasses, fast foods, soda, candy and most canned foods. RCs are quickly absorbed in your small intestine, raising your blood-sugar and blood-fat levels. Now your body must scramble to get the RCs under control before they do too much damage. At best, this is a waste of time, energy and resources. To make matters worse, the RCs in processed foods are combined with lots of fat and chemical additives.

Additives Are Better Left Out

Additives are becoming a greater problem all the time, as the number of chemical compounds dumped into our foods increases. I ask my patients to remember this simple guideline: Did Nature make the food or did man? If man made it, it's probably loaded with chemicals. Despite food-industry claims to the contrary, the overwhelming majority of these chemicals have not been properly tested. Many of them, in fact, have never been tested at all, but are allowed to remain in our food under "grandfather" clauses in the law.

Furthermore, no one has investigated to find out what happens when chemicals from different foods get together in your body. Individually, they may not be too troublesome. But when they find each other, they may combine into new, possibly harmful, forms.

I have seen many patients suffering from a variety of problems that cleared up when they stopped eating chemical-laden foods. A small number of additives may be useful for preserving freshness. The majority, however, may be not only totally unnecessary but harmful to your "doctor within."

Excess Alcohol Harms Your "Doctor Within"

Then, of course, there's alcohol. In addition to other problems we're well aware of, such as alcoholism and liver damage, drinking excessive amounts of alcohol can increase your chances of having a stroke. It is felt that alcohol harms the metabolism of the brain, heart and the blood vessels feeding the brain, increases blood pressure and sets your body to work producing more "stress" hormones. Thanks to these and other problems it causes, excessive alcohol consumption can spur you to an early grave. Don't forget, too, the 25,000 people who die on the highways and the hundreds of thousands of others who are injured in accidents involving alcohol.

How much is too much? More than one mixed drink, one can of beer or one glass of wine a day is risky for some people. Four or more mixed drinks, beers or glasses of wine is definitely a problem for everyone. Alcohol is one of life's pleasures that should be enjoyed sparingly, if at all.

Super Foods Versus the S.A.D.

The Standard American Diet is sad indeed:

Fat:	About 45% of our calories come from fat.
Protein:	About 20% of our calories come from protein.
Carbohydrates:	About 35% of our calories come from carbohydrates.

Refined Carbohydrates:	50% or more of the calories from carbohydrates come from refined carbohydrates.
Processed Foods:	75% or more of our total food intake is processed.
Cholesterol:	600 to 1,000 mg. a day.
Salt:	6,000 to 15,000 mg. a day.
Additives:	Lots.
Caffeine:	Too much.

Compare this to the Super Food Diet I've devised, which emphasizes the foods that give your "doctor within" a boost: fresh vegetables and fruits, whole grains, plus small amounts of low-fat fish, poultry, dairy products, nuts and seeds.

Fat:	About 20% of the calories come from fat.
Protein:	About 10% of the calories come from protein.
Carbohydrates:	About 70% of the calories come from carbohydrates.
Complex Carbohydrates:	Almost all of the carbohydrates are complex (little or no refined carbohydrates).
Processed Foods:	Less than 10% of our total food intake is processed.
Cholesterol:	Less than 300 mg. a day.
Salt:	300-500 mg. a day.
Additives:	As few as possible.
Caffeine:	None.

As you can see, the Super Food diet derives most of its calories from CCs, which are the best source of fuel for your body. The excess fat, protein and cholesterol, so strongly associated with many diseases, have been eliminated. Processed foods are also avoided. Of the multitude of processed foods in the typical supermarket, most are nothing more than fanciful combinations of fat, sugar, refined carbohydrates and various additives. These so-called foods are nothing more than packaged, potential disease.

Super Food Success Stories

I've used a Super Food diet as the basis of treatment for many of my patients. One woman, Sharon R., had a 20-year history of headaches. These were painful attacks on one side of her head; pounding pain accompanied by nausea and made worse by lights.

She showed me a long list of the drugs she had tried. There was aspirin, acetaminophen, codeine, Darvon and Ibuprofen. She had been put on a beta-blocker medication (Proprandol), an antidepressant and, most recently, a calcium-channel blocker (Verapamil). All these medications helped a bit but were hardly worth the side effects they caused.

After performing a thorough physical examination, ordering appropriate laboratory tests and taking a medical and personal history to rule out disease, I persuaded her to slowly reduce, then eliminate, her medications and change from her junk-food diet to a Super Food diet. Be sure to eat plenty of carrots, spinach, broccoli, cabbage, parsley, lentils and whole grains, I told her.

She did as I instructed—up to a point. She ate all the Super Foods I recommended *and* her favorite candy bars, which she insisted she could not do without. But as the days passed and she noticed that her headaches were fewer and milder, she realized that they were a reaction to the additives and sugar she was used to eating. Determined never to have another of those terrible headaches, she got rid of the candy and stuck to the Super Food diet. In the months since then, her headaches have disappeared and, as a bonus, she feels healthier and more energetic than she has in years. Oh yes, she doesn't crave candy bars anymore.

Bernice F. is another Super Food success story. She was a beautiful woman with clear, shiny skin that literally radiated health. Then she got a job as a representative for a major pharmaceutical company. Flying from city to city to put on trade conventions and meet with doctors, she ate nothing but S.A.D. hotel and restaurant food. Her diet was filled with processed foods, fatty foods, sugars and additives. Her skin became dry, and the beautiful complexion that had stopped men dead in their tracks was now pale and thick. She complained also of not being able to see well in dim light. "I must be aging," she sighed. Aging? She was only in her late 30's. "What new drug will help my skin, Dr. Fox?" she asked.

I told her she didn't need drugs, she needed carrots. She had the classic signs and symptoms of a vitamin A deficiency. But you don't need vitamin A supplements, I said. Instead, eat lots of carrots, broccoli, spinach, cantaloupes and other Super Foods rich in beta carotene. Your body will convert into vitamin A exactly as much of the beta carotene as it needs.

Bernice still travels a lot, but now she stops at a market on her way from the airport to her hotel. She buys a small bag of fresh carrots and other Super Foods, which she has the hotel keep in their refrigerator for her. She makes it a point to eat at least two carrots a day, plus as many other Super Foods as possible. Her skin has cleared up, her eyesight has returned to normal, and she's proud of the way she takes care of her "doctor within."

A Nutrition Tip from Bugs Bunny

How old is Bugs Bunny? I'm not sure, but if my memory of childhood cartoons is correct, the inimitable rabbit is probably in his 40's by now. Forty years is pretty old for a rabbit, but Bugs's "doctor within" is going strong, and he's in great shape. There are theories to explain why Bugs hasn't sickened, aged and died like regular rabbits. I can think of three:

1. He's not a real rabbit.
2. Warner Brothers won't let him.
3. He's always eating carrots.

I think number three is the real reason Bugs is so healthy. It's all those carrots he eats.

Among other things, carrots contain beta carotene, a nutrient that goes a long way toward making your immune system strong. Carotenes are pigments that give some vegetables and fruits their yellow or orange color. Green vegetables also have carotenes, but their color is masked by the green of chlorophyl.

Beta Carotene and Vitamin A

Beta carotene and the other carotenes are called "provitamin A," because they can be converted to vitamin A inside your body. Provitamin A is the plant form of vitamin A. When you eat meat, fish, dairy and poultry products, however, you take in preformed vitamin A.

I tell my patients to get most of their vitamin A from beta carotene, rather than preformed vitamin A. Why? Because to get preformed vitamin A from, let's say, meat, you're forced to swallow a lot of fat, cholesterol and who knows what chemical additives.

When you obtain beta carotene from carrots, broccoli, cantaloupes and other fruits and vegetables, however, you're eating a lot of vitamins and minerals, with only small amounts of fat and absolutely no cholesterol. Besides, the beta carotene in foods is not toxic, but large doses of vitamin A (preformed vitamin A) *may* be toxic.

Bugs Bunny isn't the only American hero who knows the value of Super Foods. Popeye is always eating spinach, which contains large amounts of beta carotene. I don't know if spinach will make your muscles grow, but I can guarantee that the beta carotene in spinach will give your "doctor within" a boost. We don't have a cartoon hero who eats sweet potatoes, but perhaps we should, because sweet potatoes are also high in beta carotene. (Sweet Potato Man?)

Beta Carotene Against Cancer

Beta carotene is a new part of cancer prevention and treatment programs. Exciting research conducted in this country and abroad indicates that beta carotene reduces the general risk of cancer in humans, especially cancer of the lungs, larynx, esophagus, stomach, colon, rectum, prostate and urinary bladder. Even if you smoke, beta carotene can help protect you against lung cancer. But please, do not use this as an excuse to smoke. There is no good reason to smoke.

Strengthening Your "Doctor Within" with Beta Carotene

Beta carotene/vitamin A is also great for your health in general. Vitamin A has long been known for its ability to protect the skin and linings (mucous membranes) of the respiratory, digestive and urinary tracts. The first line of defense against invading organisms and environmental poisons, these are very important parts of your "doctor within."

Without sufficient vitamin A, your immune system suffers. Some important parts of your immune system (thymus and lymphoid tissue) shrink, and the total number of immune-system soldiers (T-cells and B-cells) decreases, further crippling your ability to fight off disease. Because surgery normally depresses a person's immune system, I advise my patients facing surgery to boost their immune system by eating lots of beta-carotene-rich foods well before their operation.

Various studies have shown that vitamin A is especially helpful in protecting the lungs and airways. For example, the lining of the respiratory tract is destroyed in laboratory animals exposed to noxious gases. But if the animals are pretreated with vitamin A, the lining grows back.

Here's what you get* in these beta-carotene-rich Super Foods:

Nutrient (per 3 1/2 oz)	Carrots (raw)	Spinach (raw)	Sweet Potatoes (raw)
Beta Carotene	11,000.0 IU	8,100.0 IU	8,800.0 IU
Vitamin C	8.0 mg	51.0 mg	21.0 mg
Calcium	37.0 mg	93.0 mg	32.0
Phosphorous	36.0 mg	51.0 mg	47.0 mg
Iron	.7 mg	3.1 mg	.7 mg
Sodium	47.0 mg	71.0 mg	10.0 mg
Potassium	341.0 mg	470.0 mg	243.0 mg
Vitamin B_1	.06 mg	.1 mg	.1 mg
Vitamin B_2	.05 mg	.2 mg	.06 mg
Vitamin B_3	.6 mg	.6 mg	.6 mg

Notes:

mg = milligrams

IU = international units

* These and subsequent nutritional content figures are from the Agriculture Handbook No. 8 of the Consumer and Food Economics Research Division of the United States Department of Agriculture, *Composition Of Foods.*

Notice the large amounts of beta carotene in carrots, spinach and sweet potatoes. You also get healthy doses of potassium and vitamin C in raw spinach.

Crucifers Against Cancer

Crucifers are cancer-fighting Super Foods. The crucifer family includes broccoli, brussels sprouts, cabbage, cauliflower, kohlrabi and kale. Even the very conservative Committee On Diet, Nutrition and Cancer of the National Academy of Sciences agrees that crucifers, along with carrots and spinach, are important cancer fighters.

Eating crucifers encourages the formation of substances called indoles in your intestines. Studies have shown that indoles help prevent some kinds of cancer. The beta carotene, vitamin C and fiber in crucifers also work against cancer.

Besides fighting cancer, crucifers are good for your health in general. They are full of CCs but have very little fat and no cholesterol. All in all, they're just what the doctor—your "doctor within"—ordered. Broccoli is an excellent crucifer that not only supplies you with indoles and other cancer fighters but generous amounts of beta carotene and vitamin C as well.

Nutrient	Broccoli
(Per 3 1/2 oz)	(raw)
Beta Carotene	2,500.0 IU
Vitamin C	113.0 mg
Calcium	103.0 mg
Phosphorus	78.0 mg
Iron	1.1 mg
Sodium	15.0 mg
Potassium	382.0 mg
Vitamin B_1	.1 mg
Vitamin B_2	.23 mg
Vitamin B_3	.9 mg

(See notes for chart on page 43.)

Parsley: Not Just a Condiment

Parsley is a food that gets very little respect. The sprig that's set on your plate for decoration is often tossed aside. That's too bad, because parsley is surprisingly nutritious. Parsley contains a large amount of beta carotene, enough to rank it with carrots as a cancer-fighting Super Food. It also contains plenty of calcium, potassium and vitamin C. You need calcium, of course, for strong bones and for many other biochemical functions. Potassium is important for a healthy heart and for energy. When patients tell me they're tired and "don't feel well," I check their potassium level. I'm not surprised to find low levels of blood potassium in many of these patients. As for vitamin C, well, a healthy "doctor within" depends on plenty of this vitamin.

Nutrient (per 3 1/2 oz)	Parsley (raw)
Beta Carotene	8,500.0 IU
Vitamin C	172.0 mg
Calcium	203.0 mg
Phosphorus	63.0 mg
Iron	6.2 mg
Sodium	45.0 mg
Potassium	727.0 mg
Vitamin B_1	.12 mg
Vitamin B_2	.26 mg
Vitamin B_3	1.2 mg

So eat lots of parsley, the overlooked and undervalued Super Food. The little bit you occasionally find as a garnish isn't nearly enough. My wife buys it by the bunch, washes it and refrigerates it. I munch on it whole or chop it up and toss it in my salad.

Orange Fruits Put You in the Pink of Health

Here are three foods you may not have thought were Super Foods: cantaloupes, papayas and peaches. These orange fruits contain large amounts of beta carotene; cantaloupes and papayas also contain quite a bit of vitamin C.

Nutrient (Per 3 1/2 oz)	Cantaloupe (raw)	Papaya (raw)	Peach (raw)
Beta Carotene	3,400.0 IU	1,750.0 IU	1,330.0 IU
Vitamin C	33.0 mg	56.0 mg	7.0 mg
Calcium	14.0 mg	20.0 mg	9.0 mg
Phosphorus	16.0 mg	16.0 mg	19.0 mg
Iron	.4 mg	.3 mg	.5 mg
Sodium	12.0 mg	3.0 mg	1.0 mg
Potassium	251.0 mg	234.0 mg	202.0 mg
Vitamin B_1	.04 mg	.04 mg	.02 mg

Vitamin B_2	.03 mg	.04 mg	.05 mg
Vitamin B_3	.6 mg	.3 mg	1.0 mg

(See notes for chart on page 43.)

Papayas should be eaten when they're soft but still firm. And cantaloupes should be eaten plain, without sugar. "But it won't taste sweet without the sugar, Dr. Fox," some of my patients have complained. We've gotten so used to dumping sugar on everything that we don't realize how sweet some foods naturally are. So leave the sugar off. Your taste buds will tell you what a sweet-tasting melon it is all by itself.

Hot and Spicy Super Foods

As an internist and cardiologist, I've seen many patients die when a blood clot lodges in a narrow artery in their heart, choking off the flow of blood and triggering a heart attack. Inappropriate blood clots can cause all kinds of trouble. Former President Nixon was put on blood thinning drugs to prevent unwanted blood clots. But why wait until after the heart attack or stroke has occurred? Wouldn't it be better to prevent dangerous clots from forming in the first place?

Garlic is a spicy Super Food that works against heart disease by helping to prevent these dangerous blood clots from forming. The oil in garlic tends to prevent platelets in the blood from clumping together and becoming blood clots. Garlic oil also helps to break up clots that have already formed. Studies have indicated that garlic oil also reduces cholesterol and triglyceride (fat) levels in the blood.

If you have coronary artery disease, or want to avoid it, mixing garlic with your food is helpful. If you don't like garlic, try onions, scallions (green onions), ginger or black Chinese mushrooms, all of which have anticlotting properties.

Fibrous Super Foods

Legumes, whole grains and oat bran are Super Foods that help us fight both cancer and heart disease.

We're all familiar with the whole grains: buckwheat, barley, millet, whole wheat, whole-grain rye, brown rice and others. Legumes are peas, beans and lentils. Which peas and beans? All of them are Super Foods except soybeans, which are higher in fat. They include: kidney beans, lima beans, navy beans, pinto beans, white beans, garbanzos (chick peas), red beans, peas, split peas, snow peas, English peas and more.

The Standard American Diet emphasizes meat, dairy products and refined foods, leaving little room for whole grains, peas, beans and lentils. The grains we do eat are refined, which means they've been stripped of their nutritive value and turned into the RCs (refined carbohydrates) that shock your "doctor within" with excess energy. When we do eat beans, they are generally swimming in a sugary sauce mixed with fatty pork and chemicals. And lentils, well, many people don't even know what lentils are. It's too bad the S.A.D. overlooks legumes and whole grains, for they offer a lot of fiber that can really help your "doctor within."

Oat Bran Versus Cholesterol

Oat bran is one of my favorite Super-Food grains. I recommend it to all my patients who want to protect themselves against a heart attack. My own studies indicate that, in addition to lowering overall cholesterol levels, oat bran helps raise your HDL—high-density lipoprotein—the "good cholesterol" that helps keep arteries clear.

Practically every patient I see for the first time has a high cholesterol level. This puts them at greater risk for heart disease. There are medications to lower cholesterol, and sometimes they must be used. But these drugs, like all drugs, have dangerous side effects. I usually put my patients on a low-fat, low-cholesterol, high-CC diet, which lowers their cholesterol better than the drugs do, without any side effects other than better all-around health.

I once pitted a Super Food diet rich in oat bran against a cholesterol-lowering drug. Two of my patients had been on the medication for several months. The first patient's cholesterol had actually risen a bit. So had his LDL—low-density lipoprotein—"bad cholesterol."

I placed these same two patients on the low-fat, low-cholesterol, low-sugar, Super Food diet, with special instructions to eat 1/2 cup of oat bran in the morning and three oat-bran muffins a day. In three months I measured their cholesterol levels again. In both patients cholesterol levels had dropped from dangerously high to reasonably safe. (I like to see cholesterol below 180. Under 160 is excellent.) The ideal figure is 100 plus your age.

Cholesterol	Beginning Level	Ending Level
Patient #1	247	180
Patient #2	260	190

I also checked their HDL and LDL levels. (I tell my patients to raise their HDL to 50 or higher, and get their LDL down to 100 or less.)

	Beginning Level	Ending Level
HDL ("good cholesterol")		
Patient #1	35	50
Patient #2	28	55
LDL ("bad cholesterol")		
Patient #1	176	105
Patient #2	255	135

The Super Food diet, with added oat bran, did a better job than the cholesterol lowering drugs, without any side effects. No side effects, that is, except for giving their "doctor within" plenty of nutrients to use in building vibrant health.

Oat bran lowers cholesterol by increasing the excretion of bile acids in the stool. (Bile acids, which are made in your liver, are used to absorb fat in your food, and some are partially reused to make cholesterol.) Eating oat bran helps you excrete as much as 50 percent more bile acid than you normally would. Greater excretion of bile results in less cholesterol.

Oat bran isn't the only food that lowers blood cholesterol. Grains, beans, lentils and other fibrous foods all protect against heart disease by lowering cholesterol.

Fiber Beats Cancer, Intestinal Disorders, Diabetes

Fibrous Super Foods are especially helpful in fighting cancer and intestinal disorders. Eating a lot of fiber makes your stool bulkier and softer, pushing it rapidly through the bowels. Getting the stool out faster reduces the amount of time your gut lining is exposed to potential carcinogens in the stool. In addition, fiber promotes the growth of aerobic bacteria (bacteria that requires oxygen to live) in the intestines, rather than the anaerobic bacteria encouraged by the low-fiber S.A.D. The S.A.D.'s anaerobic bacteria can break down bile acids into cancer-causing substances.

Thanks to the large amounts of fiber in my Super Food diet, straining and constipation are eliminated. This protects against hemorrhoids, appendicitis, varicose veins, diverticulosis (weak pockets in the large intestine caused by straining and constipation) and diverticulitis (an inflammation of those weak pockets). Gastroesophageal hiatal hernia, a condition that allows acid to pour onto the lining of the esophagus and cause the common "heartburn," is also greatly ameliorated by the fibrous Super Food diet.

I've found fiber-rich diets to be useful in combating both insulin-dependent and noninsulin-dependent diabetes. Most of my diabetic patients who have given up the S.A.D. in favor of a Super Food diet rich in fibrous foods have been able to reduce the amount of insulin they must take. Many can eventually do without insulin altogether.

High-fiber diets have another benefit: they can help you lose weight. Since we don't digest and absorb fiber, it adds no calories to our diet. It also gives us a full feeling, so we don't rush right back to the refrigerator after a meal.

Fiber, the Cinderella Food

Fiber used to be scorned as peasant food. Today, from Beverly Hills to Park Avenue, people appreciate the health value of fiber and are finding more ways to add it to their diets. The Super Food peas, beans, lentils and whole grains, are good sources of fiber. Kidney beans, lima beans, navy beans, pinto beans and white beans are unusually rich sources of fiber.

Moderately good sources of fiber include: whole-wheat bread and pasta, oatmeal, chick peas, lentils, artichokes, asparagus, green beans, brussels sprouts, red and white cabbage, carrots, cauliflower, corn, green peas, kale, parsnips, potatoes, spinach, celery, tomatoes, apples, apricots, bananas, cantaloupes, blueberries, cherries, grapefruits, oranges, peaches, pears, pineapples, raisins and strawberries. Popcorn is also a fairly good source of fiber, but be sure to eat it plain, without added butter and salt.

Sweet Red Peppers and Other Uncommon Super Foods

"I know what red peppers are, but what are beet greens, collards and kale?" That's the typical reaction to my suggestion that people start eating these overlooked Super Foods. You'll find beet greens, collards and kale in the vegetable section of your market. They're the foods you walk right by, hardly noticing, as you head for the more familiar spinach and lettuce.

In addition to large amounts of beta carotene and potassium, beet greens, collards and kale contain good supplies of vitamin C. Sweet red peppers are great sources of vitamin C and beta carotene.

There is no doubt that the immune systems suffers if it doesn't get enough vitamin C. Patients with low levels of vitamin C in their blood (hypoascorbemia) not only suffer from retarded wound healing, they are able to mount only weak defenses against invading microbes. The ability of the immune system to fight back depends on sufficient amounts of this important vitamin.

I like to dice up these Super Foods, rich in beta carotene and vitamin C, and add them to my daily salad.

Nutrient (Per 3 1/2 oz)	Beet greens (raw)	Collards (raw)	Kale (raw)	Sweet Red Peppers (raw)
Beta carotene	6,100.0 IU	9,300.0 IU	10,000.0 IU	4,450.0 IU
Vitamin C	30.0 mg	152.0 mg	186.0 mg	204.0 mg
Calcium	119.0 mg	250.0 mg	249.0 mg	13.0 mg
Phosphorus	40.0 mg	82.0 mg	93.0 mg	30.0 mg
Iron	3.3 mg	1.5 mg	2.7 mg	.6 mg
Sodium	130.0 mg	— mg	75.0 mg	— mg
Potassium	570.0 mg	450.0 mg	378.0 mg	— mg
Vitamin B_1	.1 mg	.16 mg	.16 mg	.08 mg
Vitamin B_2	.22 mg	.31 mg	.26 mg	.08 mg
Vitamin B_3	.4 mg	1.7 mg	2.1 mg	.5 mg

(See notes for chart on page 43.)

Wet Your Whistle with a Liquid Super Food

Be good to your body. Give it lots of water. Not coffee or soda or hot chocolate, but water. Men's bodies are approximately 60 percent water; women's are about 50 percent water. Our bloodstream is watery; our cells are filled with and surrounded by water; our muscles contain plenty of water, and our brain has even more. Even our hard, solid bones are full of water.

We lose a lot of our water every day: in urine, feces and sweat. A little more water is lost with the air we exhale. A person can live 100 or more days without eating, but only five to ten days without replenishing the body's supply of water.

So, pure water is an excellent Super Food. It has no fat, cholesterol or calories—just the H_2O your body needs. I tell my patients to drink six to eight, eight-ounce glasses of water each day.

Super Food Round-Up

Here, then, are the Super Foods, each with its one or more special, health-building properties:

Beans	Collards	Peaches
Beet Greens	Garlic	Peas
Black Chinese		
Mushrooms	Ginger	Sweet Red Pepper
Broccoli	Kale	Scallions
Brussels Sprouts	Lentils	Spinach
Cabbage	Oat Bran	Sweet Potatoes
Cantaloupes	Onions	Water
Carrots	Papayas	Whole Grains
Cauliflower	Parsley	

The ideal food would be full of CCs, vitamins, minerals and fiber, with just enough protein and a little bit of fat. Unfortunately, the perfect food does not exist. Even the Super Foods, good as they are, have their limitations. Carrots, for example, have plenty of beta carotene and potassium but very little vitamin C. Red peppers are rich in vitamins C and A but have little calcium. White beans have a good amount of calcium but no vitamin A. The best approach, then, is to eat a wide variety of Super Foods.

I usually put my patients on a diet that strongly emphasizes a broad spectrum of Super Foods, depending on their unique health status. Those who are at high risk for heart disease, for example, should eat a lot of fibrous Super Foods to help lower their cholesterol, plus garlic, onions, ginger or black Chinese mushrooms to assist in controlling unwanted blood clots.

The point is to give their "doctor within" the strength needed to repair their body and regain good health. As their health improves, I have my patients broaden their diet to include many other nutritious foods. These may not be on the same high health level as Super Foods, but they're good for you and your "doctor within."

Choosing foods for the Super Food diet is simplicity itself. Simply go to the produce section of your market and fill your basket with fresh vegetables, beans, peas and fruits. Next, select dried or sprouted beans, peas and lentils. Then go to the shelves where the whole grains are kept. Be sure to get whole-grain rice, not white rice. Remember the general rule: Did Nature make the food or did man? Nature creates whole-grain rice and whole wheat. You can also purchase grains such as barley, millet and cracked wheat. Or look for breads, rolls and pasta made from whole wheat and other whole-grain flours. Add low-fat fish to your shopping basket, along with your favorite herbs and spices.

When Less Is More

When it comes to eating meat, less is more. If you feel you must have meat, select the very lean cuts and eat only a little, to flavor the other foods. As Thomas Jefferson said: "I attribute my longevity to the fact that I use meat as a condiment, not as an aliment." Poultry and dairy products should also be eaten with restraint. Chicken has less fat, but it contains almost as much cholesterol as red meat. Buy small amounts of white chicken. Be sure to remove the skin before cooking, and prepare and eat your chicken without oils and/or fatty sauces.

Dairy products contain bone-building calcium; unfortunately, they also have plenty of fat and cholesterol.

So always look for the low- or non-fat varieties, such as uncreamed cottage cheese made from hoop cheese. Nuts and seeds add flavor and nutrition to your diet, but they should be used sparingly because they are high in fat.

What to Eat?

I tell my patients to fill their kitchens with these Super Foods and other healthy foods (Super Foods are starred):

VEGETABLES

Artichokes	Chard	*Parsley
Asparagus	Cucumbers	Parsnips
*Beet Greens	Eggplant	Potatoes
Beets	*Garlic	Radishes
*Black	*Ginger	Rutabagas
Chinese	Green	*Scallions
Mushrooms	Peppers	*Spinach
*Broccoli	Jicama	Squash
*Brussels	Kohlrabi	*Sweet
Sprouts	Leeks	Potatoes
*Cabbage	Lettuce	*Sweet Red
*Carrots	Mushrooms	Peppers
*Cauliflower	Okra	Watercress
Celery	*Onions	Zucchini

- Vegetables are low in fat, sugar and sodium and contain no cholesterol. Vegetables provide you with complex carbohydrates, fiber, vitamins, minerals and enzymes.
- Eat more raw than cooked vegetables. Cooking destroys many nutrients.
- Instead of boiling or baking vegetables, steam them—just until they're tender, yet crisp. Steamed vegetables are tasty and nutritious.

FRUITS

Apples	Figs	*Peaches
Apricots	Grapes	Pears
Bananas	Guavas	Persimmons
Berries	Mangoes	Pineapples
*Cantaloupes	Melons	Plums
Cherries	Oranges	Pomegranates
Citrus Fruits	*Papayas	Tomatoes

- Fruits are low in fat and sodium and contain no cholesterol. Fruits provide vitamins, minerals and sweetness.
- Uncooked, unprocessed, fresh fruit should be your first choice, rather than canned, cooked or frozen.

WHOLE GRAINS

* Barley	* Millet	* Whole-Grain Rye
* Brown Rice	* Oat Bran	* Whole-Grain Wheat
* Buckwheat	* Whole-Grain Oats	* Wild Rice

- Whole grains are low in fat, sugar and sodium, and contain no cholesterol. Whole grains give you complex carbohydrates, fiber, B vitamins, minerals and low-fat protein.
- Make sure to eat *unprocessed* whole grains rather than processed grains such as white rice and white bread.
- Oat bran is not a whole grain. I've listed it with the whole grains because of its cholesterol-lowering effects, plus its high fiber content.

LEGUMES

* Black Beans	* Kidney Beans	* Pinto Beans
* English Peas	* Lentils	* Red Beans
* Garbanzo Beans	* Lima Beans	* Snow Peas
(Chick Peas)	* Navy Beans	* White Beans
* Green Beans	* Peas	

- Legumes are low in fat, sugar and sodium, and contain no cholesterol. Legumes provide you complex carbohydrates, fiber, low-fat protein, vitamin B_1, vitamin B_6, calcium, iron, plus other vitamins and minerals.

FISH

Abalone	Halibut	Sea Bass
Brook Trout	Red Snapper	Sole
Cod	Sand Dabs	Tuna
		(packed in water)
Flounder	Scallops	Yellow Perch
Haddock		

- The fish listed above are low-fat fish.
- Shellfish, such as crabs, lobster and clams, are not high in fat, but people trying to lower their cholesterol should eat them sparingly or not at all.
- Fish are a good source of protein.
- Broil or steam your fish. Cooking and/or serving in oils or rich sauces adds lots of fat.
- Eat tuna fresh or, if canned, packed in water, not oil. Six percent of the calories in tuna packed in water are fat, but an astounding 60 percent of the calories in tuna packed in oil are fat. * Mussels and oysters have fair amounts of fat, so limit your consumption of these shellfish.
- Recent studies in medical journals have shown that even a small intake of fish, one or two meals a week, reduced the incidence of coronary heart disease.
- Certain fish, such as salmon, herring and mackerel, have a protective effect against heart disease even though they are higher in fat than the fish listed above. It's felt that a special kind of fatty acid, called omega-3, confers the protective effect. Here's a list of fish high in omega-3 fatty acids (modified from the *Journal of the American Dietetic Association*):

Fish (3 1/2 ounces)	Grams of Omega-3
Sardines, Norway	5.10
Salmon, Chinook	3.04
Mackerel, Atlantic	2.18
Pink Salmon	1.87
Albacore Tuna (canned, light)	1.69
Sablefish	1.39
Herring, Atlantic	1.09

Rainbow Trout	1.08
Pacific Oyster	.84
Striped Bass	.64
Channel Catfish	.61
Alaskan King Crabs	.57
Ocean Perch	.51
Halibut, Pacific	.45
Shrimp	.39
Flounder, Yellowtail	.30
Haddock	.16

- For my patients who are at risk for coronary artery disease (those with elevated cholesterol, blood pressure or triglycerides or those with known coronary artery disease), I recommend three to four servings of fish a week. Of those meals, two or more should be fish high in omega-3s.

FOWL

	% of Calories From Fat
Chicken (white meat)	15
Chicken (dark meat)	32
Turkey (white meat)	20
Turkey (dark meat)	37

- As you can see, the white meat of chicken is low in fat and falls well within the fat guideline for the Super Food diet. The dark meat of chicken, and the white and dark meat of turkey, are also relatively low in fat (compared to red meat).
- 3 1/2 ounces of uncooked chicken contain 60 mg. of cholesterol. The average amount of cholesterol in 3 1/2 ounces of uncooked beef is roughly 70 mg. You can see that although chicken is much lower in fat than beef is, there isn't an appreciable difference between the two when it comes to cholesterol. So eating lots of chicken isn't a good way to lower your cholesterol.
- Eat white-meat chicken and turkey, cooked after the skin has been removed.

- Steam or broil your chicken and turkey. Cooking and/ or serving in rich sauces or oils adds lots of fat.
- Chicken and turkey provide protein, vitamins and minerals.

DAIRY PRODUCTS

	% of Calories From Fat
Regular Milk	47
Low-Fat	30
Skim (Nonfat)	2

- As you can see, regular milk is high in fat. But because milk is such a good source of dietary calcium, I tell my patients to drink skim milk (if they have no intolerance to it).
- Many adults can't drink milk because they have what is known as lactose intolerance. They lack an enzyme called lactase, which digests lactose (milk sugar).
- Cheese is made from milk. The type of milk used to make the cheese determines how fatty the cheese will be. Most common cheeses are made from regular milk. Because cheese has much less water than milk, the percent of calories from fat in cheese is much higher than in milk.

	% of Calories From Fat
Cheddar	71
Swiss	67
Blue (Roquefort)	73
Parmesan	58
Cottage cheese, Creamed	35

- Hoop cheese (also know as farmer's cheese) is a very low-fat cheese made from skim milk. It gets only about 3 percent of its calories from fat.
- If you like yogurt, eat the unsalted nonfat skim milk type. Or you can easily make your own nonfat yogurt.
- Dairy products provide no fiber.
- Here are some nonfat and low-fat cheeses:

Nonfat Cheeses
  Ricotta (all skim milk)
  Washed Cottage-Cheese Curd
  Fromage Blanc (white cheese, French)

Very Low-Fat Cheeses
  Fromage Fort (Canquillote) Farmers (German)
  Gammelost (Blue Mold)   Sap Sago
  Bakers   St. Otho
  Danish Export

Moderately Low-Fat Cheeses
  Feta (imported)   Finnish Jack
  Mozzerella   Parmesan
  Edam   Imported Swiss
  Danbo   Neufchatel
  Tybo   Port du Salut
  Jarlsburg

NUTS AND SEEDS

Nuts:
Almonds   Hazelnuts   Pecans
Chestnuts   Macadamias   Walnuts
Filberts

Seeds:
Anise   Dill   Sesame
Caraway   Flax   Sunflower
Chia   Poppy   Pumpkin
Celery

- Nuts and seeds are high in fat, deriving about 70 percent to 87 percent of their calories from fat (depending on the nut). Use them sparingly. Macadamias contain the highest percentage of calories from fat. Chestnuts, which are very low in fat, are an exception, and roasted chestnuts taste great.
- If you use nuts and seeds, use them sparingly as a condiment, to give your food extra taste and crunch.

SPICES

Anise	Dillweed	Oregano
Basil	Dill Seed	*Parsley
Bay Leaves	Dry Mustard	Pepper
Cardamom	*Garlic (fresh)	Paprika
Cayenne Pepper	*Ginger	Rosemary
Celery Seeds	Horseradish	Soy Sauces
Cinnamon	(powder)	(low salt)
Cloves	Mace	Thyme
Coriander	Marjoram	Vanilla Extract
Cumin (ground)	Nutmeg	White Vinegar
Curry Powder	Onion Powder	

Enemies of Your "Doctor Within"

As you go through your market selecting Super Foods and other healthy foods, you'll find yourself bypassing the majority of items on the shelves. These are the processed foods and junk foods, the enemies of our "doctor within."

If you carefully read the labels, you'll find that many packaged, canned and frozen items have very little real food left in them, and even less real food value. Many of their nutrients have been heated, frozen, processed or leached out. What you get is the food "shell," along with large dollops of added fat, salt, sugar and chemicals. Occasionally, you also receive just enough spray-on vitamins to satisfy government regulations.

Nature fills her foods with nutrients. Man fills his foods with fat, sugar, salt, fillers, modifiers, texturizers, flavors, preservatives and coloring agents. I am awed by the creativity of food chemists, but I am alarmed by their lack of concern for our health.

Compare a real potato, for example, to a typical brand of artificially flavored mashed potatoes. A potato contains potato. Artificially flavored mashed potatoes contain potato flakes, monoglycerides, natural and artificial flavors, sodium bisulfite, calcium stearoyllactylate, BHA and BHT, sodium acid pyrophosphate and citric acid. Now, I'm not saying that everything in artificial potatoes is harmful. But why take a chance when the alternative is a tasty, 100 percent safe and nutritious potato? It comes back to the general rule: Did Nature make the food or did man? Nature makes potatoes. Man makes artificial potatoes.

Fast foods are also a health problem, for the same reason that processed foods are. The people who make fast foods and processed foods load their products with fat, sugar, refined carbohydrates, salt and chemical additives.

When Is a Potato Chip Not a Potato Chip?

Let's look at the potato again. A potato baked in its skin is full of complex carbohydrates; it contains vitamins, minerals and a little bit of protein and fat. Less than one percent of its calories come from fat. When you turn it into a French fry, it gets 40 percent of its calories from fat. By the time it becomes a potato chip, it gets a whopping 64 percent of its calories from fat. It's not a potato chip, it's a fat chip! The CCs and nutrients are mostly gone, replaced by fat, salt and chemicals.

Unfortunately, the same scenario is repeated over and over with fast food. For example, fairly healthy, low-fat chicken becomes fatty, salty, processed chicken, served in a white-flour bun full of RCs and flavored with sugary ketchup.

Refined foods, processed foods and junk foods are incomparable sources of fat, sugar, RCs, salt and chemical additives. That's bad news for you and your "doctor within."

A Note on "Diet"

The Super Food diet isn't the type of diet you go on for two weeks or two months and then stop. It's not a weight-loss diet that you stop when you've lost enough pounds, or a "health" diet you eat until you feel better. The Super Food diet is a blueprint for healthy living. It's a game plan, a lifelong approach to keeping your "doctor within" hale and hearty. Make the Super Food diet part of your everyday life.

What About Supplements?

"Well, eating Super Foods makes sense to me, but what about vitamins and minerals? Should I take supplements?" Some people claim that we don't need to take vitamin and mineral supplements if we're eating a "good" diet that supplies all the RDAs (Recommended Dietary Allowances).

Unfortunately, relatively few of us eat a "good" diet. Studies have shown that most people aren't taking in all the RDAs. But even consuming all the RDAs won't guarantee good health. Why? Because the RDAs are set much too low. They're based on the dangerous either/or approach to health: you're either sick or you're healthy. If you don't have scurvy or another of the classic vitamin-deficiency diseases, then you're getting all the vitamins you need. As we've seen, however, the either/or approach to health is an invitation to trouble.

You don't wake up one morning to find yourself suddenly suffering from a serious vitamin-deficiency disease. Instead, your nutrient status gradually slips from healthful to terrible, with signs and symptoms sounding warnings along the way.

Very few of us can boast of having all the vitamins, minerals and other nutrients we need for optimum health. Most of us are lacking in several vitamins and minerals. Our body tries to tell us that something is wrong, but we don't recognize the signs and symptoms.

I believe that problems related to lack of nutrients are relatively common. But our medical system doesn't consider nutrient deficiencies to be a problem; not until they produce an obvious disease. Recurrent infections and personality changes, for example, simply do not qualify.

So millions of people are left to suffer, wondering why they're sick or unhappy so often. They don't know that their problems are related to nutrient deficiencies, but they do know that they don't feel right.

It's only when a person has a recognizable disease that doctors begin to pay serious attention. Now the patient has a disease that can be labeled. But which disease? A lack of vitamins and minerals can prompt immune-system malfunctions that can result in any number of diseases, from the mild to the very serious.

Nutrition for Your Immune System

Is the deficit of a vitamin or two all that harmful? After all, you never hear of anyone in this country dying from a lack of vitamin C or iron. Death certificates rarely state that the cause of death was nutrient deficiency. But as a physician I can tell you that many illnesses and deaths are caused by, or related to, nutrient imbalances. It may be lack of certain vitamins and minerals, or it may be excess fat, cholesterol or sugar that's the culprit. A shortage or excess of even one nutrient can knock your immune system off balance. While your immune system totters, you're more susceptible to disease. I've treated thousands of patients whose problems were related to a nutrient-starved immune system.

Bs on the Brain

Nutritional deficiencies can attack your immune system directly, or they can launch a two-stage attack by way of the mind. Lack of nutrients, especially the B vitamins, can lead to such personality changes as depression, irritability, nervousness, anxiety and moodiness. As a group, the B vitamins are especially important for maintaining a positive outlook on life.

As we learned earlier, there are physical and chemical links between mind and body. What kind of thoughts will an anxious, depressed, irritable mind generate? The kind that harm the "doctor within" and the immune system. That's why it's important to take in plenty of the nutrients that will keep you happy.

Nutrition profoundly influences your immune system, both by direct action and by way of the mind.

Many Factors Affect Your Nutrient Requirements

Let's suppose you eat an abundance of Super Foods, that your diet is filled with vitamins and minerals significantly above the RDAs. Do you need to take supplements?

How many vitamins and minerals you consume is only one side of the equation; your nutrient requirement is the other. There are many factors that increase your need for vitamins and minerals. Alcohol, coffee, tea, tobacco, marijuana, refined foods and radiation, for example, lower the blood levels of one or more B vitamins. Premenstrual tension lowers the blood level of vitamin E. Physical and emotional stress increases your need for vitamin C, the B vitamins and zinc. Air pollution increases your need for vitamin C.

Many common medicines interfere with the absorption of the vitamins and minerals you eat or prevent your body from utilizing them properly. Aspirin, mineral oil, antacids, oral contraceptives, antibiotics, diuretics, pain medications and heart medications can increase your nutrient requirements.

Nutri-Prevention

I feel that almost everyone could benefit from a program of supplements. I call the supplement programs I've developed for my patients Nutri-Prevention—the use of nutrients to prevent disease.

I'm not advocating vitamin and mineral pills as the cure for any and all problems. In conjunction with the Super Food diet and the rest of the Immune for Life program, however, Nutri- Prevention can add a great deal to your health and happiness.

Don't rush out to a health food store and buy a shopping bag full of vitamins and minerals. In the Immune for Life Workbook section, you will be taking three quizzes. Your scores on these quizzes will indicate which of the four Nutri-Prevention supplement programs in Chapter Eight may be best suited to your needs.

The Immune for Life menus and recipes in the next chapter, meanwhile, will show you how to make Super Foods and other healthy foods the basis of a delicious daily diet.

Chapter 3

Immune for Life Menus and Recipes

Leave gourmandizing. Know the grave doth gape for thee
thrice wider than for other men.
                                    Shakespeare, Henry IV, Part I

*B*ut Dr. Fox, some patients complain, "Food
is so much fun! It's my only enjoyment in life." I answer
that food and eating should always be pleasurable, but
food and eating are not, and should not be, the sole
enjoyment in life. Life has a great deal else to offer: love,
friendship, beauty, nature, knowledge, humor, explora-
tion, the joy of nurturing, the excitement of pursuing a
goal, the thrill of physical activity and sport, the satisfaction
of quiet contemplation.

Food can be, and should be, a sensual delight.
Ironically, most of us don't know what food tastes like.
We know the taste of fat, sugar and salt, in all their many
combinations, but we are largely unfamiliar with the taste
of real food.

The Immune for Life philosophy states that food is
a very pleasurable necessity of life. It tastes great and
gives you a comfortable, full feeling in your stomach. But
food is also the raw material our "doctor within" uses
to build health, happiness and longevity. That means we

must eat good-tasting foods that also boost our "doctor within."

Choose your foods from the abundance of great-tasting fresh fruits, vegetables, whole grains and whole-grain breads, rolls and pastas that are available. Low-fat fish is delicious, as is fish that is high in omega-3s. Small amounts of nonfat or low-fat poultry and dairy products add even more variety. With spices, herbs and small amounts of nuts and seeds, you can create innumerable taste sensations.

The first step is to decide that you want to live young and healthy to a very old age. Then make a point of discovering all the wonderful tastes the Standard American Diet overlooks. Be adventurous. Try eating vegetables raw or lightly steamed, not boiled to death or hidden under mounds of butter and sauce. Learn what food, all by itself, without added salt, sugar and fat, really tastes like. Find out how much zest garlic, ginger, herbs and spices add to food.

The recipes that follow will give you an idea of the different ways to prepare healthy foods. Some I created, and others were given to me by my patients, friends and family. I encourage you to experiment until you figure out exactly what you like and how you like it prepared. Feel free to add or subtract ingredients, alter the instructions or invent your own dishes. Super Food cooking isn't the type of gourmet cooking that requires precise measurements and timing. In fact, on many recipes I simply say "spice to taste," because I want you to turn cooking into a discovery process.

VEGETABLE DISHES

NO-OIL SAUTE

Many recipes call for sauteed foods. To saute without oil, get a frying pan large enough to hold whatever you're going to cook, then add 1/4 cup water and put over a medium heat. When the water is boiling, place the food in the pan and quickly move it around, using a wooden spoon or other implement to turn it on all sides, until the outside is very lightly cooked.

SANDWICH-BAG VEGETABLES

Many of us are so accustomed to eating boiled, soggy vegetables that we don't realize many fresh vegetables taste great raw. They're cool, crisp and crunchy.

I tell my patients to carry a sandwich bag full of fresh vegetables with them during the day for lunch, dinner or snacks. Fill the bag with any fresh raw vegetables you like, such as carrots, celery, spinach, lettuce, snow peas, green beans, sprouts, broccoli, cabbage, cucumbers, cauliflower, beet greens, chard, jicama, leeks, mushrooms, okra, parsley, red peppers, watercress, zucchini or any other vegetables you choose.

STEAMED VEGETABLES

For a quick, easy-to-prepare entree or side dish, simply wash your favorite vegetables, and place them in a steamer. Steam lightly, so vegetables are crisp and tasty. How long you steam each vegetable depends on your taste.

Lightly steamed food is generally more nutritious than foods cooked in other ways. With steaming, there aren't the high temperatures or cooking oil that destroy and leach nutrients out of the food.

My favorite vegetables for steaming include carrots, broccoli, cabbage, spinach, mushrooms, sweet potatoes, brussels sprouts, corn and cauliflower.

I put all the vegetables in the steamer at once and steam them together for 10 to 15 minutes. I use a double-decker steamer, putting the lighter, quicker-cooking vegetables on top and the heavier ones on the lower level.

BAKED POTATO

A baked potato is a nutritious, low-calorie dish that's easy to prepare. Preheat oven to 400. Wash and dry the potato; puncture it several times with a fork. Place on baking sheet, tinfoil or oven rack and bake for approximately

45 minutes, or until soft. (Cooking time depends on size of potato and your taste.)

Don't add butter, sour cream, cheese or other fattening toppings to your potato. Eat it plain or sprinkle on chives, parsley, mint, basil, nonfat yogurt or one of the dressings on pages 97–100. Believe me, try it and you'll love it just this way.

Another tasty way to prepare potatoes is to steam or bake a potato, then cut it into 1/2″ slices. Put the slices on a nonstick pan and bake in the oven.

SPINACH LASAGNA
    1 lb. whole-wheat lasagna noodles
    2 bunches spinach
    1 lb. hoop cheese
    1 32 oz. can tomato sauce (no salt added)
        spices to taste

Boil and drain noodles. Wash and chop spinach and mix with hoop cheese. Thinly cover bottom of a large baking dish with the tomato sauce. Place a layer of noodles over the tomato sauce, then a layer of spinach and cheese, then another layer of sauce. Repeat until baking dish is filled. Make sure a layer of sauce is on top. If you like, sprinkle top with diced green peppers and shaved carrots. Bake 30-40 minutes at 350°.

Serves 6 to 8.

PITA SANDWICH
Fill pita bread with sprouts, diced tomato and cucumber, chopped onions, some garlic and a tablespoon of low-fat cottage cheese.

HERBED VEGETABLE SAUTE
    1 celery stalk
    1 onion
    1 sweet red pepper
    1 cup broccoli florets

      2 carrots
1/4 lb. mushrooms
1/2 clove garlic, minced
  3 cups brown rice, cooked
           lemon juice
           spices to taste
           1/4 cup sunflower and sesame seeds
           parsley

Wash all vegetables. Chop celery, onion, red pepper and broccoli, slice carrots and mushrooms. In water, saute garlic, celery, onion, red peppers, carrots, broccoli and mushrooms. Add cooked rice and a little water to skillet; cover and let sit for a few minutes. Season to taste; garnish with parsley. Sprinkle with lemon juice and seeds, and serve.

Serves 3.

GARLIC CARROTS
  1/2 cup parsley
     2 lbs. carrots
   2 large garlic cloves, pressed
  1/2 cup water
2-3 tbls. vinegar
  1/8 tsp. cayenne pepper
  1/2 tsp. paprika
  1/2 tsp. cumin powder
           parsley

Wash carrots and parsley. Chop parsley; peel and slice carrots. Put carrots, water and garlic in shallow pan of water, and simmer until just tender. Save cooking liquid for stock. Put carrots on plate; cover with vinegar, cayenne, paprika, and cumin. Garnish with parsley. Serve cold.

Serves 6 to 8.

SUNSET BOULEVARD CARROTS
          2 cups brown rice, cooked
          2 cups barley, cooked
           1 lb. carrots
          2 cups Mama Fox's Spaghetti Sauce (see page 95)
                  several sprigs parsley

While Mama Fox's Spaghetti Sauce, brown rice and barley are cooking, lightly steam and dice carrots. When everything is ready, mix brown rice and barley, spread over bottom of dish. Put carrots over the grains, pour spaghetti sauce over carrots. Season to taste, garnish with parsley.

Serves 4.

SOUTH PHILLY VEGGIE DIP
     1/2 bunch parsley, minced
            1 onion, chopped
       3 cups garbanzo beans, cooked
      2/3 cup sesame seeds
     1/2 tsp. oregano
        1 tsp basil
               dash of cumin
               dash of garlic powder

Wash and mince parsley. Saute onion in water. Blend or mash garbanzo beans with all other ingredients. Use as a dip for raw vegetables or a sandwich spread.

Makes approximately 5 cups.

CRUNCHY POTATO SALAD
         2 lbs. potatoes
       1/2 cup celery
       1/2 cup sweet red peppers
       3/4 cup scallions
       1/4 cup parsley
       1/2 cup nonfat yogurt

2 tbls. cider vinegar
1 tsp. curry powder

Wash all vegetables. Skin potatoes, chop celery, pepper
and parsley; thinly slice scallions. Steam or boil potatoes
until tender, then drain. Cut potatoes into 1/2-inch cubes,
and combine with chopped vegetables. In a small bowl,
mix yogurt, vinegar and curry powder. Stir yogurt
mixture into potato mixture. Cover and refrigerate until
serving time. Excellent for carry-out lunches.

Serves 4 to 6.

OKRA STEW
        1 large onion
        4 medium tomatoes
1 clove garlic, minced
        1 six-oz. can tomato paste
2 tsps. lemon juice
1/2 tsp. oregano
1 lb. okra

Wash vegetables. Chop onion and tomatoes. Saute onion
and garlic in water until tender. Add tomato paste,
tomatoes, lemon juice and oregano. Cover and simmer
for 20 minutes. Wash okra and cut off the cone-shaped
top. Add to tomato mixture. Simmer, covered, 20-30
minutes. Serve over hot grains.

Serves 4.

SALADS

A salad is anything you want it to be. I've been served
salads that consisted of 10 or 12 different sliced and
chopped vegetables on a bed of spinach and lettuce. I've
also eaten salads that were nothing more than a few slices
of cucumber, one cherry tomato and a piece of iceberg
lettuce.

I tell my patients to include at least four or five different kinds of vegetables in their salads. Which? My favorites are carrots, broccoli, cabbage, parsley, tomatoes, spinach, kale, collards, beet greens and onions. There's also lettuce, cauliflower, jicama, mushrooms, cucumbers, celery, red and green peppers, okra, squash, radishes, sprouted peas, sprouted beans and sprouted lentils.

You can prepare the vegetables any way you like, from chopping them into big pieces to shredding them in a food processor. What do you top a salad with? Raisins, a few sunflower seeds or nuts, lemon juice or other fruit juice. But don't ruin a healthy salad by covering it with fatty, sugary or oily dressings—that defeats the purpose. Special low-fat, low-sugar dressings are OK. Vinegar is also fine, if it's not mixed with oil.

Fruit salads are mixtures of fresh fruits. You can eat a fruit salad as is, or with raisins or perhaps a few sunflower seeds. I like to chop up the fruit and mix it with low-fat cottage cheese, nonfat, plain yogurt, or Fairfax Hoop Dressing.

With these notes on salads in mind, here are some salad recipes:

DR. FOX'S SUPER SALAD

      1 2-inch wide slice of cabbage
      2 leaves collards, large
    1/3 cucumber, medium size
     10 string beans
    1/3 sweet red pepper
      2 carrots, medium size
    1/4 onion, white or purple, medium size
      1 clove garlic
      2 tsps. sunflower seeds
        white pepper
        cumin
      2 ozs. tuna, packed in water
        vinegar

This recipe requires a food processor. Wash all vegetables. Slice the ends off string beans. Crush garlic clove. Using shredding blade, shred all vegetables and garlic in food processor. Add sunflower seeds and toss. Add cumin and white pepper to taste. Break tuna into small flakes and sprinkle over the salad. Add vinegar to taste, and serve.

Try making this salad in different ways. Sometimes I use pineapple chunks instead of tuna and pineapple juice instead of vinegar. Or, try it with a tablespoon of low-fat cottage cheese instead of tuna.

Serves 2.

CRUCIFER AND CARROT SLAW SALAD
      1 cup carrots, shredded
      1 cup cabbage, shredded
      1 cup cauliflower, shredded
      1 cup broccoli, shredded
      2 apples, diced
  1/2 cup cucumbers, sliced
  1/4 cup slivered almonds, raw

Toss and serve. If you like, make a dressing by pureeing 1 banana with 1/2 cup buttermilk and 1/4 cup hoop cheese in a blender.

Serves 4 to 6.

POTPOURRI SALAD
  1 1/2 cups cabbage, shredded
      1 cup carrots, shredded
      1 cup celery thinly sliced
      1 cup white turnips, thinly sliced
      1 cup cauliflower, thinly sliced
      1 cup broccoli stalks, thinly sliced
  1/2 cup radishes, thinly sliced
  3 or 4 broccoli florets for decoration
              parsley

Arrange vegetables, except broccoli florets and parsley, in separate mounds on a serving platter. Decorate with broccoli florets and parsley.

Serves 5 to 6.

L.A. SPROUT SALAD
    1 cup lentil sprouts
    1 cup mung or azuki bean sprouts
    1 cup alfalfa sprouts
    1 cup celery, chopped
        1 apple, chopped
        2 scallions, chopped

Combine ingredients, mix and serve.

Serves 4 to 6.

BEVERLY HILLS COLESLAW
    4 cups cabbage, thinly sliced
    3/4 cup celery, thinly sliced
    3/4 cup fresh pineapple, thinly sliced
    2/3 cup scallions, thinly sliced
    1 small sweet red pepper, thinly sliced

Mix ingredients and serve.

Serves 4 to 6.

CAROTENE SALAD
    4 large carrots, grated
    1 cup spinach, shredded
    1/4 cup watercress
        1 scallion, chopped
        3 oranges, peeled, and diced
    1/2 cup radishes, sliced

Combine ingredients, mix and serve.

Serves 4 to 6.

EASTERN SALAD
    1 cup ripe tomatoes, chopped
    1 cup green apple, diced
    1 cup onion, chopped
    1 cup green pepper, seeded, diced
    2 tsps. hot green chili pepper, seeded, finely
            chopped
    6 tbls. vinegar or lemon juice
    1 tbl. dried mint leaves, pulverized

Combine all vegetables and apple in a bowl. Add vinegar, mint, mix and serve.

Serves 4 to 6.

LEGUMES

MIXED SPROUTS AND RAISINS

Sprouted beans and peas are tasty, high in vitamin C, and add crunch to your foods. Buy mixed sprouts (or sprout your own), including mung bean sprouts, azuki bean sprouts, lentil sprouts, pea sprouts and radish sprouts.

Fill a small bowl with the mixed sprouts. Add raisins to taste. Sprinkle with sunflower seeds or chopped peanuts or almonds. Eat and enjoy. My son Barry likes to eat mixed sprouts and raisins with a small slice of low-fat mozzarella cheese and a piece of whole-wheat bread.

MIXED BEANS

Mixed beans, with or without lentils, can be eaten by themselves or as part of a meal. My wife Hannah always keeps a big pot of six or seven kinds of cooked beans in the refrigerator, ready to be heated or eaten cold as part of a salad.

How long it takes beans to cook depends on whether, and how long, you presoak them. To presoak beans, rinse them, and then place in a pot with about three times as much water as beans. Let stand for several hours. When my wife cooks beans, she puts them in a pot with three cups of water for every cup of beans. She puts the slower-cooking beans in first, adding the quicker-cooking ones a little later. The water is brought to a boil, the beans are added, covered, and left to simmer over a low heat. She checks the water occasionally, adding more if necessary.

Here are approximate cooking times for beans:

Bean (one cup)	Hours cooking	Water	Yield
Black Beans	1 1/2	4 cups	2 cups
Black-eyed Peas	1	3 cups	2 cups
Garbanzo Beans	3	4 cups	2 cups
Kidney beans	1 1/2	3 cups	2 cups
Lentils	1	3 cups	2 1/4 cups
Lima Beans	1 1/2	2 cups	1 1/4 cups
Navy Beans	1 1/2	3 cups	2 cups
Pinto Beans	2 1/2	3 cups	2 cups
Split Peas	1	3 cups	2 1/4 cups
White Beans	1 1/2	3 cups	2 cups

GREEN BEAN CECY

- 1/4 cup green pepper
- 1/4 cup sweet red pepper
- 1/2 cup celery
- 1 1-lb. can tomatoes (no salt added)
- 1 lb. fresh green beans
- 1/4 lb. fresh snow peas
- 1/2 tsp. onion powder

Wash all vegetables. Dice green and red peppers. Thinly slice celery. Crush tomatoes. Steam green beans until tender, then combine in pot with other ingredients. Cook over medium heat for 10 minutes.

Serves 6 to 8.

WILSHIRE BARLEY BEAN
        1 carrot, large
        1 onion, large
        2 stalks celery
        1 potato, large
  1/2 cup pearled barley
  1/2 cup lima beans, large
           white pepper
           garlic powder

Wash all vegetables. Dice carrot and onion, thinly slice celery. Cut potato into medium-size pieces. Put barley and beans into a 3-quart pot. Fill with water to cover beans and barley by an inch. Bring barley and beans to a boil, then reduce to simmer. Cook 20 minutes, then add other ingredients; cook until lima beans are tender. Add water if necessary.

Serves 4 to 6.

BEAN SALAD
     1/2 cup mixed beans and lentils, cooked
        1/2 tomato
  2 1/4 inch onion slices
      1 tsp. salsa (no sugar added)
  1/2 clove fresh garlic, minced

Mix all ingredients and enjoy.

Serves 1.

PETY'S CHILI
    2 cups kidney beans, raw
  1/2 cup small white beans (navy)

        1/4 cup yellow split peas
          1 cup raw bulgar
              1 onion, chopped
      4 cloves garlic, crushed
          1 cup carrots, chopped
          1 cup celery, chopped
                 white pepper, chili powder and garlic
          1 cup sweet red peppers, chopped
    2 1/2 cups fresh tomatoes, chopped
        5 tbls. tomato paste
                 juice of 1/2 lemon

Cook beans and peas in 2 quarts of water until tender, (about 1 hour), adding more water if necessary. Boil 2 cups water in pot, add raw bulgar, cover pot and let stand for 15 minutes while bulgar cooks. Saute onions and garlic in water. Add carrots, celery and spices. When vegetables are almost done, add peppers, tomato paste and lemon juice. Cook until tender. Combine all ingredients and heat together gently in moderate oven. Serve topped with low-fat Parmesan cheese and parsley.

Serves 6 to 8.

BEAN LENTIL SUPREME
        1/2 cup dried white beans
        1/2 cup lentils
        1/2 lb. cabbage
              4 carrots
              3 stalks celery
        1/2 lb. Chinese mushrooms
              3 tomatoes
              2 potatoes
              2 onions, chopped
      2 cloves garlic, minced
         6 cups water
         1 tsp. tomato paste
              8 slices whole-wheat bread
                 white pepper to taste

Cook beans and lentils separately, as suggested on page 78. Save cooking water. In blender or food processor, puree half the beans and lentils. Set aside.

Wash all vegetables. Core and shred cabbage, grate carrots, chop celery, slice mushrooms, peel and chop tomatoes and dice potatoes. Saute onions, garlic, carrots and celery in water. Add cooking water, plus enough water to make 6 cups, tomatoes, tomato paste, remaining vegetables, seasonings, beans, pureed beans and more water if necessary. Bring to a boil, reduce heat and simmer about 1 hour.

Toast bread, break into croutons. Mix soup and bread pieces in bowls; garnish with chopped green onions and parsley.

Serves 8.

MARGARITA'S BLACK BEANS AND RICE
            1 onion
            1 sweet red pepper
    1 clove garlic
       2 qts. water or stock
       1 lb. black beans
       1 tsp. oregano
            1 bay leaf
     2 tbls. cider vinegar
     1 cup brown rice, cooked
              a pinch of cayenne pepper

Slice onion, dice pepper and crush garlic. Cook all ingredients, except rice, together for 3 hours, or until beans are tender. Serve over 1 cup cooked brown rice. Garnish with tomato wedges, chopped green onions and chopped parsley.

Serves 6 to 8.

FISH

STEAMED FISH

Steaming is a very simple way to prepare fish. Simply put the low-fat fish into a closed sandwich bag and place in a steamer. Steam until tender, remove from sandwich bag and eat. This is one of my favorite ways to prepare fish. The fish cooks in its own natural juice; no oil or butter are added. And there's no mess to clean up.

An easy way to prepare a tasty and healthy meal is to steam fish, cut into small pieces, and mix with brown rice and barley. Season as you desire. I like to flavor it with garlic and parsley.

FLIPPER'S CHOICE

       1 lb. low fat fish fillets
              pepper
              garlic powder
              basil
              oregano
              onion powder
       1   sweet red pepper
       1   can tomato sauce (no salt added)

Wash and dry fish fillets, cut into 2-inch strips. Place in baking dish; sprinkle on all the spices. Wash and slice red pepper, and place slices on top of fish. Pour tomato sauce over fish. Bake 10 minutes at 375° without turning.

Serves 2.

MILK FISH

       4 6-oz. snapper or perch fillet
   1/2 cup nonfat milk
            tarragon
            dillweed
            onion powder
            paprika

Preheat broiler. Dip fillets in milk, place in shallow baking dish and sprinkle with tarragon, dillweed, onion powder and paprika to taste. Broil about 3 inches from the heat source for 3 to 4 minutes, basting once with drippings. Turn, baste and sprinkle with additional herbs if desired. Broil 3 to 4 minutes longer.

Serves 4.

PASSYUNK FISH
        2 onions
        2 lemons
        3 garlic cloves, minced
        1 cup celery
        1 small eggplant
        1 large tomato
        1 small can tomato paste, with water to make 1
           1/2 cups
           1/2 tsp. cumin
   1/2 lbs. low fat fish

Preheat oven to 350. Wash vegetables. Thinly slice onion and lemon, chop garlic buds and celery, dice eggplant and slice tomato. Use a heavy pan to saute onions and garlic in water. Add celery and eggplant, tomato paste, water and spices. Cook about 10 minutes. Spread half the resulting sauce in a baking dish, put in fish; top off with remaining sauce, lemon and tomato slices. Cover dish and bake about 20 minutes. Uncover; cook 5 minutes more. Serve with brown rice.

Serves 2 to 3.

TUNA SPROUTS
        8 stalks celery
        2 large onions
   4 ozs. fresh mushrooms
    1 cup homemade chicken broth
           garlic powder

1 tsp. salt-free soy sauce
2 tbls. cornstarch
1 cup water
1 6.oz. can bamboo shoots
2 cups fresh bean sprouts (any kind)
7 ozs. tuna (water packed, drained, preferably no
salt added)
2 cups brown rice or barley, cooked pepper

Wash vegetables, cut celery diagonally, thinly slice onions and slice mushrooms. Place chicken broth in a covered pot, and add garlic and soy sauce. Heat over medium heat until simmering. Stir in cornstarch until dissolved, cover pot and and set aside. Heat 1/3 cup water in wok over high heat. Stir-fry celery and onion in wok for 1 minute. Add bamboo shoots, mushrooms and sprouts, continue stir-frying for additional minute. Add broth mixture and cook until sauce is thickened, mixing frequently. Add tuna and stir. Serve immediately over brown rice or cooked barley.

Serves 2 to 3.

MAY'S SALMON (OR TUNA) PATTIES
2 large cans red or pink salmon (skin, bones
removed)
OR
4 7-oz. cans tuna (packed in water)
6 egg whites, beaten with fork
1/2 cup matzo meal (without salt) or whole-wheat
bread crumbs
1/3 tsp. white pepper
1/3 tsp. garlic powder
4 scallions
parsley sprigs

Crumble salmon (or tuna), mash with fork. Add egg whites, matzo meal, white pepper and garlic powder; mix well. Form mixture into 8 patties, and place on baking sheet sprayed with Pam. Bake for 1/2 hour in 350° oven. Wash and chop scallions, and sprinkle on top. Serve topped with Yogurt-Garlic Dressing (page 100); sprinkle with fresh-cut parsely.

Serves 4 to 6.

CHICKEN

Before cooking chicken, regardless of the recipe, cut away the skin and all visible fat. Be sure to remove the skin before cooking, before the fat seeps from the skin into the chicken.

CHICKEN BOUILLON
         4 chicken breasts
       2 qts. water
     1/3 tsp. garlic powder
     1/4 tsp. white pepper

Remove the skin and all visible fat from the chicken breasts. Place in large pot with water and bring to a boil. Let boil 2 minutes, reduce heat to medium. Add garlic powder and white pepper. Cook 2 minutes more, stirring constantly. Then, put on low heat and cook for 30 minutes. Remove chicken from liquid, and let liquid cool. Skim fat off the top.

The liquid is your chicken bouillon to use in other recipes. Slice the chicken breasts and use in sandwiches, or dice and combine with minced celery and cucumber, pureed in a blender, and you have a chicken salad.

Makes 2 quarts.

SIMPLE BAKED CHICKEN
         1 chicken breast
       1 cup applesauce (approximately)
             apple or pineapple juice (optional)

For a quick, simple, chicken dinner, cut away the skin and all visible fat from chicken breast. Coat the bottom of a pan with applesauce (no sugar added), about 1/4 inch high. Put chicken in pan, and bake at 350° until tender. If you like, you can pour a little apple or pineapple juice over the chicken before you bake it.

Serves 1.

CHICKEN RATATOUILLE
       1 lb. mushrooms
       1 lb. eggplant
   1/2 lb. zucchini
       1 lb. tomatoes
       4 chicken breasts
    1 tsp. white pepper
       1 bay leaf
    2 tsp. onion powder
    1 tsp. garlic powder
    1 tsp. oregano, crumbled

Cut mushrooms into halves, eggplant and zucchini into 3-x-1 inch fingers. Slice and crush tomatoes, keeping pieces and juice together. Skin chicken, cut away visible fat and sprinkle both sides with white pepper. Place chicken in shallow roasting pan or large, ovenproof skillet. Bake at 450° for 20 minutes, or until lightly browned. Remove chicken and pour off drippings. Reduce oven temperature to 350°. In roasting pan, combine undrained tomatoes, eggplant, zucchini, mushrooms, bay leaf, onion and garlic powders and oregano. Place chicken breasts on top of vegetable mixture, spooning some of the sauce over breasts. Cover and bake 30 minutes. Uncover and bake until chicken is fork-tender, about 15 minutes.

Serves 4.

CHICKEN AND RED PEPPER RICE
<pre>
    1 sweet red pepper
    2 whole green scallions
  1/2 garlic clove
1/4 cup chicken bouillon (more if necessary)
 4 oz. chicken, diced
1/2 cup brown rice, cooked parsley
1/4 cup Mama Fox's Spaghetti Sauce (optional)
</pre>

Wash and chop red pepper. Wash and chop scallions into small sections, setting aside green parts. Crush garlic. Saute the crushed garlic and sliced scallions in chicken bouillon for 2 to 3 minutes. Bring to a high heat and add chicken. Cook for 2 to 3 minutes, stirring frequently. Lower heat and simmer until chicken is tender. Add cooked brown rice and chopped red pepper. Toss until rice is coated with sauted mixture. Top with scallion tops and parsley and serve. I like to pour some of Mama Fox's Spaghetti Sauce over my Chicken and Red Pepper Rice.

Serves 1 to 2.

CHICKEN ARIBA
<pre>
    4 potatoes, medium
    1 onion, large
    2 carrots, large
1/2 lb. green beans
    2 chicken breasts, split
 2 cups fresh corn kernels
         garlic powder
         white pepper
         parsley
         sunflower seeds
</pre>

Preheat oven to 350°. Slice peeled potatoes in 1/2-inch sections. Peel onion and slice thickly. Peel carrots, quarter lengthwise and cut into 2-inch strips. Cut ends off the green beans. Remove skin and visible fat from chicken. Place chicken in pot, saute in water or chicken broth for

5 minutes. Then, place onions on top of chicken and other vegetables, including corn, on top of onions. Season with garlic powder and pepper. Cover and bake for 40 to 60 minutes, or until vegetables and chicken are tender. Garnish with parsley and sunflower seeds.

Serves 4.

ROBIN'S PINEAPPLE CHICKEN AND RICE
              1 chicken, cut-up
      1/2-3/4 fresh, or 1 can sliced pineapple (in own juice)
      1/2 cup slivered almonds (no salt added)
      1/2 cup raisins
        1 cup brown rice

Remove skin and visible fat from chicken, place in pan. Slice 1/2 to 3/4 of fresh pineapple into medium size slices, saving juice. Pour raisins and almonds over chicken, place fresh or canned pineapple slices on chicken, pour pineapple juice over chicken. Bake chicken at 350° for 1 hour, or until chicken is brown. Cook rice while chicken is baking. When chicken and rice are ready, remove the pineapple slices from chicken, cut into small pieces, add to rice. Remove 1/2 the raisins and almonds and some of the pineapple juice from chicken, add to rice. Serve chicken with remaining raisins and almonds in dish with rice mixture.

Serves 3 to 4.

GRAINS
OAT BRAN

A bowl of oat bran in the morning is a great way to start the day. You get fiber and complex carbohydrates, plus oat bran's anti-cholesterol power. You can eat oat bran by itself, or mixed with oatmeal or other grains. I like a mixture of oat bran and Scottish oats, seasoned with a little cinnamon powder. Sometimes I add just a little apple juice for a different taste.

To cook oat bran, bring 1 cup of water to a boil, stir in 1/2 cup of oat bran. Cook over low heat for 5 to 10 minutes, or to taste. Stir occasionally, watch closely and add water if necessary.

OATMEAL

Like oat bran, oatmeal is great by itself or mixed with other grains. Use old-fashioned oats or raw oats from a health food store. Stay away from precooked oats. Experiment with the different varieties of oatmeal and find the one you like best.

To cook oatmeal, bring 1 cup of water to a boil, stir in 1/2 cup of oatmeal. Cook over low heat for 3 to 5 minutes, or to taste. Stir occasionally, and add water if necessary. If you like a dryer, firmer oatmeal, cook for just a few minutes over a higher heat, stirring frequently. If you like a more souplike oatmeal, use more water and cook longer. Try mixing your oatmeal with cornmeal or couscous.

BROWN RICE, BARLEY AND OTHER GRAINS

Alone, mixed, or added to other foods, whole grains make a tasty, nutritious meal. A bowl of grain can be the basis for a meal. Just add a little bit of chicken or fish, along with your favorite seasonings. Mixed grains with steamed vegetables is a great high-fiber, low fat, no-cholesterol meal.

To cook grains, bring water to a boil and stir in grain. Let water boil again, then reduce heat to simmer and cover. Check water level occasionally, adding more if necessary.

Grain (one cup)	Cups water	Minutes cooking	Yield
Barley, Pearled	3	40	3 1/2 cups
Brown Rice	2	60	3 cups
Bulgur Wheat	2	15	2 1/2 cups

Grain (one cup)	Cups water	Minutes cooking	Yield
Coarse Cornmeal (Polenta)	4	25	3 cups
Couscous ("Moroccan Pasta")	2	10	2 cups
Kasha (Buckwheat)	2	15	2 1/2 cups
Millet	3	45	3 1/2 cups
Whole-wheat Berries	3	120	2 2/3 cups

One of my favorite dishes is a mixture of brown rice, barley and couscous with pressed garlic and a few sesame seeds. It's a nutritious, high-fiber, low-fat taste treat.

SPROUT AND RICE SALAD

        1 sweet red pepper
        1 scallion
        1 carrot
   2 cups brown rice, cooked, cooled
  1/2 cup lentil sprouts
  1/2 cup mung bean sprouts
  1/2 cup azuki bean sprouts
  1/4 cup sunflower seeds, raw, unsalted
  1/4 cup raisins
           several sprigs parsley

Clean vegetables. Chop red pepper and scallions, and grate carrot. Spread cooked rice evenly on a dish. Mix the sprouts, sunflower seeds and vegetables in a bowl, then spoon over rice. Sprinkle with raisins, and garnish with parsley.

Serves 4.

SAUTEED CARROTS AND ONION IN BARLEY AND MILLET

            1 onion
          1/2 carrot
    2 cloves garlic, minced
      1 cup barley, cooked
      1 cup millet, cooked
    1/4 cup raisins
              dash of cayenne pepper

Wash vegetables. Chop onion and shred carrot. Saute onions and garlic in water. Mix barley, millet and raisins in a bowl; add onions, garlic and carrot. Season with cayenne pepper, or other spices, to taste.

Serves 2.

KASHA (BUCKWHEAT) AND FISH

Here's a tasty and wholesome meal that's easy to prepare.

    2 cups kasha
    6 ozs. low fat fish
            garlic powder
            white pepper
            lemon juice
            curry powder

Cook the kasha (see page 89). Steam fish (see page 82). When fish and kasha are ready, fork-cut fish into small pieces and mix with kasha. Season with garlic powder, white pepper and lemon juice, and/or curry powder. If you prefer, use rice, barley or other whole grains.

Serves 2.

MIDDLE EAST RICE OR MILLET

    2 cups brown rice or millet
    2 tbls. sesame seeds

>   2 tbls. raisins
>   1 tbl. lemon juice

Cook brown rice or millet (see page 89). Add other ingredients, mix and serve.

Serves 2.

YOGURT MILLET OR RICE

>   2 cups brown rice or millet
>   2 cups plain yogurt
>   2 tbls. fresh ginger, finely chopped
>   1/2 sweet red pepper, diced
>   1 tsp. celery seeds

Cook brown rice or millet (see page 89). Add other ingredients, mix and serve.

Serves 2.

SOUPS

STOCK

Whenever you steam or cook vegetables, save the water to use as stock in soups. Store in a covered glass jar in refrigerator.

BETA CAROTENE FRUIT SOUP

>   1 banana
>   2 apricots
>   1/4 fresh cantaloupe
>   1 papaya
>   1 peach
>   1 lemon
>   1 cup low-fat yogurt
>   3 cups unsweetened, unfiltered apple juice

Peel and chop the banana, apple, apricots, cantaloupe, papaya and peach. Squeeze juice from the lemon into a cup and discard rind. Place all ingredients in blender and blend until thick and creamy. If you prefer soup thicker, add more banana. If you prefer it thinner, add more fruit juice. Chill and pour into soup bowls, or mix with crushed ice and drink. Top with parsley.

Serves 5.

VEGETABLE SOUP

3	carrots
1/2 lb.	string beans
1	onion, large
1	potato, large
1/4 head	cabbage
8	okra (optional)
6	mushrooms, large
2	ears fresh corn
1	tomato, large
3 stalks	celery
1	zucchini, large
2/3 cup	brown rice
1 lb.	green peas, shelled
	garlic powder
	white pepper

Clean and/or peel all vegetables. Slice carrots into 1-inch pieces. Cut ends off string beans, then cut in half. Slice onion. Dice potato into large pieces. Shred cabbage. Slice okra and mushrooms. Use knife to remove kernels from corn cobs. Dice tomato. Slice celery into 1/4-inch pieces. Slice zucchini into 1/2-inch strips. Cook rice in water for about 1/2 hour, until half cooked, then set aside. In a large Dutch oven, saute onions, tomato, celery and mushrooms for 3 minutes, stirring constantly. Add garlic powder and white pepper to taste. Add two quarts water, bring to a boil; add brown rice, string beans, corn and carrots. Cook over medium heat for 20 minutes. Add potato, cabbage, okra, peas, zucchini (and more water if necessary); simmer an additional 20 minutes.

Serves 4 to 6.

SHIRLEY'S ZUCCHINI SOUP
         2 lbs. zucchini
            3 onions
       4 cups chicken stock
       1/2 cup skim milk
         1 tsp. curry powder

Cut zucchini into 1/4 inch slices. Thinly slice onions. Put zucchini and onion slices in stock, and cook until very tender, about 20 minutes. Puree vegetables and stock in blender. Add 1/2 cup skim milk and curry powder to taste. Serve warm or chilled. Makes a thick, tasty soup.

Serves 3 to 4.

VEGETABLE BARLEY SOUP
            3 carrots
     1 bunch broccoli
            3 potatoes, medium
            2 tomatoes, medium
            1 onion, finely chopped
       1/2 cup barley
       3 cups water or chicken stock
         1 tsp. basil
         1 tsp. oregano
       1/4 tsp. dill
         1 tsp. vegetable seasoning
                  pinch of chopped parsley
                  pinch of chopped mint

Wash vegetables. Slice carrots, cut broccoli into small pieces and dice potatoes and tomatoes. Set aside. Saute onion, put in pot with barley and water (or stock) and bring the mixture to a boil. Then reduce the heat and simmer until the barley is almost done, about 30 minutes. Add the vegetables and spices; continue simmering until the vegetables are tender. Check water while soup is simmering; add more if necessary. Add the fresh parsley and mint just before serving.

Serves 4 to 6.

SPAGHETTI SAUCE
MAMA FOX'S SPAGHETTI SAUCE

        1 onion
      6-8 mushrooms
        2 zucchini
  3 cloves garlic, crushed
    1 tsp. olive oil
  1-15 oz. can peeled tomatoes (no salt or sugar added)
  1/3 cup red wine
           oregano to taste

Wash and chop onion, mushrooms and zucchini. Saute garlic, onion and zucchini in olive oil. When zucchini is almost soft, add mushrooms. Saute 2 to 3 minutes, or until vegetables are cooked to taste. Add tomatoes, wine and oregano. Use a spoon to gently break up tomatoes. Bring to a boil, reduce heat and let simmer until thick. Add water as necessary. Serve over wholewheat pasta or whole grains.

Makes approximately 3 cups.

YOGURT DISHES

Here are a few recipes I devised after buying some nonfat yogurt at the market. These are my favorite kinds of recipes: no cooking and no measurements. Nonfat (skim milk) yogurt is preferred because of its low fat content.

HOMEMADE STRAWBERRY YOGURT
  1 handful plus 6-8 strawberries, fresh
  16-oz. container yogurt, plain, nonfat

Crush a handful of strawberries to get the juice, or juice them lightly in a blender. Strain juice from pulp and reserve. Slice 6 to 8 strawberries into thin slices. Mix the sliced strawberries and yogurt in a dish. Pour the strawberry juice over the mixture. Eat chilled.

If you prefer, use apples, bananas, oranges or any other fruit.

Serves 1.

RODEO AND WILSHIRE YOGURT

The combination of ingredients is unusual, but I really like it.

> 1 tomato
> 1 peach, peeled
> 1 handful uncooked oatmeal
> 1 6 oz. container yogurt, plain, nonfat

Wash and dice the tomato and peach; mix with yogurt and oatmeal. Eat chilled. Unconventional, but nutritious and tasty. This also works well with a pear, a peach or with a dash of vanilla extract. Why is it called "Rodeo and Wilshire"? Because that's one of my favorite corners in Beverly Hills.

Serves 1.

DR. FOX'S FAVORITE

> 1/2 cucumber
> 1 6-oz. container yogurt, plain, low fat or nonfat
> cumin, to taste
> white pepper

Dice half of a chilled cucumber and mix into a bowl with yogurt. Sprinkle cumin and a pinch of white pepper over the top. Eat chilled.

Serves 1.

TOMATO TUNA COTTAGE CHEESE

> 2 tomatoes
> 3 slices onion
> 4 tsps. tuna
> 3 tbls. cottage cheese, low.fat

3 tsps. Mama Fox's Spaghetti Sauce
           cumin (optional)
           curry powder (optional)

Dice onions and tomatoes, break tuna into flakes and combine with cottage cheese and spaghetti sauce. Try adding a pinch of cumin and curry powder.

Serves 1.

DRESSINGS FOR RAW VEGETABLES, COOKED VEGETABLES AND SALADS

TOMATO—YOGURT SALAD DRESSING

    1 cup tomato puree
    1 cup yogurt, plain, nonfat
    1 tbl. cider or wine vinegar
    1 tbl. dry mustard
    1 tsp. dill weed
    2 tsps. lemon juice

Combine all ingredients and puree in blender or food processor.

Makes 3 cups.

FAIRFAX HOOP DRESSING

    1/2 cup hoop cheese
    1/2 cup buttermilk
        1 scallion, chopped
        juice of 1 lemon
    2 tsp. dill weed
        1 garlic clove
    1/2 tsp. thyme

Combine all ingredients and puree in blender or food processor.

Makes 2 cups.

BLENDER BROCCOLI DRESSING
>1 cup broccoli florets, steamed until tender 1/4 cup
>   cider or wine vinegar
>1 tbl. tomato paste
>   pinch of basil
>   dash of dill weed
>   dash of cumin
>   dash of pepper

Combine all ingredients and puree in blender or food processor.

Makes 2 cups.

NO OIL DRESSING
>   8 ozs. tomato sauce
>   2 tbls. tarragon vinegar
>   1 tsp. Worcestershire sauce
>   1 tsp. Angostura Bitters
>   1/2 tsp. dill weed, dried
>   1/2 tsp. basil, dried crushed
>   1 tbl. onion, diced
>   2 cloves garlic, minced
>   1 1-inch long chili pepper, ground

Combine all ingredients and puree in blender or food processor until smooth.

Makes 2 cups.

TOMATO HERB DRESSING
>   8 ozs. tomato juice
> 1 1/2 tbls. lemon juice
>   1/2 tbl. vinegar
>   1 tsp. Worcestershire sauce
>   1 tsp. onion juice
>   2 cloves garlic, crushed
>   2 drops Tabasco sauce
>   1/2 tsp. dry mustard

> 1 tsp. herb mix (choose some or all: rosemary, thyme, basil, coriander, cassia, mustard seed, oregano, fennel)

Combine all ingredients and puree in blender or food processor until smooth.

Make 2 cups.

RUSSIAN DRESSING
> 1 cup cottage cheese, low fat
> 1 tbl. vinegar or lemon juice
> 1/4 cup tomato juice
> 1/4 cup celery, finely chopped

Put cottage cheese, vinegar or lemon juice, and tomato juice in blender. Blend until smooth, adding more tomato juice if necessary. Stir in celery just before using.

Makes 2 cups.

YOGURT-GARLIC DRESSING
> 1 cup yogurt, plain, nonfat
> 1 1/2 tsps. cumin seeds, crushed
> 1/2 tsp. curry powder
> 1/2 clove garlic, pressed

Combine all ingredients and puree in blender or food processor.

Makes 2 cups.

HEALTHY PUREE
> 1 cauliflower
> 1/2 cup yogurt, plain, nonfat
> 1/2 bunch fresh dill or cilantro, chopped

Steam cauliflower until tender; coursely chop. Puree with yogurt in blender. Mix in fresh dill or cilantro. Serve on baked tomatoes, cooked grains or fish.

Makes 2 to 3 cups.

SPICES

Here are some of the herbs and spices you can use to add zest to your foods. I've indicated how I like to use them. Experiment and discover how they can best please your palate.

Allspice—combines well with other spices; use in vegetable dishes and dishes with tomato sauce.

Anise—use on raw vegetables.

Basil—use in vegetables dishes, soups, salads, chicken and fish dishes.

Bay Leaves—use in soups and fish dishes.

Caraway Seeds—use in vegetable and grain dishes.

Celery Seeds—use in vegetable and fish dishes, salads, soups.

Cinnamon—use in vegetable and grain dishes. Great with oatmeal and oat bran.

Coriander—use in bean dishes.

Cumin—use in vegetable dishes, soups.

Curry Powder—a mixture of cumin, ginger, coriander, turmeric, pepper, nutmeg and other spices. Use in many dishes.

Dill—use in vegetable, fish and chicken dishes, soups and salads.

Fennel—use in vegetable and fish dishes, salads and soups.

Garlic—use this Super Food in a variety of vegetable, grain, chicken and fish dishes. Great with oatmeal and oat bran.

Horseradish—grated, not prepared; use in fish dishes.

Marjoram—use in salads, vegetables and fish dishes, and dishes with tomato sauce.

Mint—use in fish dishes, vegetable and fruit salads.

Oregano—use in dishes with tomato sauce, salads and bean dishes.

Rosemary—use in poultry, vegetable and pasta dishes.

Sage—use in vegetable and chicken dishes.

Thyme—use in fish and vegetable dishes.

Turmeric—use in fish and rice dishes.

MENUS

Here are two weeks' worth of menus that will give you an idea of the many healthful combinations of meals that can be prepared. These menus are not rigid formulas. As long as you eat lots of Super Foods, a wide variety of other healthy foods, and small amounts of low-fat dairy products, fish, poultry, nuts and seeds, you'll do all right.

I haven't indicated how large each serving is because this isn't a weight-loss or weight-gain diet. The serving size depends on your appetite. The menus simply show you some of the different possible combinations of healthy foods. These menus aren't written in stone; feel free to experiment. Since the point is to eat a variety of foods, a meal composed of several small servings is fine.

WATER— Water is a vital daily nutrient. I tell my patients to drink 64 ounces of water every day. That comes out to eight, 8-ounce glasses or four, 16-ounce glasses of water a day. Drink water with every meal, as well as at other times during the day.

SNACKS— Snacks are fine as long as they are healthy foods. I suggest a carrot for a snack every afternoon. Carrots taste great, have plenty of beta carotene and other nutrients, but contain no cholesterol and only a little fat. Other raw vegetables are also good.

BREAKFAST

My idea of a good breakfast is a whole-grain cereal, a glass of skim (nonfat) milk and a fresh fruit. Whole grain cereal has generous amounts of complex carbohydrates, which give you a steady stream of energy throughout the morning. Skim milk is a good source of calcium, an important nutrient. You can drink it or pour it over your cereal. Any fresh fruit is fine. You can eat it whole or slice it into your cereal.

CEREALS

Oat bran
Oatmeal (my favorite is Irish oatmeal)
Whole-grain cereal—look for a 5- or 7-grain cereal
Rice, barley, kasha, couscous or other grains from the
pot of grains you keep in the refrigerator.
Corn meal
    You can eat the grains or cereals plain, with your
skim milk or with fruit, cinnamon, raisins, a few sunflower
seeds, a little fruit juice, or low-fat yogurt. Use your
imagination, but keep it healthy.

TWO WEEKS OF
LUNCH AND DINNER

Day 1

Lunch: Fruit salad
        Whole-wheat bread
        Cold, sliced, sweet potatoes

Dinner: Steamed fish
         Steamed crucifers
         Side of kasha
         Wedge of lettuce with sliced tomatoes

Day 2

Lunch: Sandwich-Bag Vegetables
        Whole-wheat tortilla
        Sprouts
        Plain yogurt
        Fruit

Dinner: Mama Fox's Spaghetti Sauce
         Whole-wheat pasta
         Romaine lettuce, cucumber, tomato,
         radishes

Day 3

Lunch: Mixed Sprouts and Raisins

Whole-wheat pasta (leftover)
1/2 papaya or an apple

Dinner: Simple Baked Chicken
Vegetable and Barley Soup
Dr. Fox's Super Salad

Day 4

Lunch: Homemade Strawberry Yogurt
Whole wheat bread
1/2 melon or grapefruit

Dinner: Flippers's Choice
Baked potato
Eastern Salad

Day 5

Lunch: Pita Sandwich
Fruit
Sandwich-Bag Vegetables

Dinner: Pety's Chili with bread
Zucchini Soup
Sliced tomato and cucumber
Fruit

Day 6

Lunch: Dr. Fox's Favorite
Sandwich-Bag Vegetables
1/2 melon or grapefruit

Dinner: Spinach Lasagna
L.A. Sprout Salad
Fruit Salad

Day 7

Lunch: Fruit Salad
Whole-wheat bread
Sandwich-Bag Vegetables

Dinner: Passyunk Fish
Steamed Vegetables
Dr. Fox's Super Salad
Cucumber and carrots

Day 8

Lunch: Tomato-Tuna Cottage Cheese
Banana
Whole-wheat bread

Dinner: Robin's Pineapple Chicken and Rice
Green Bean Cecy
Sliced apple

Day 9

Lunch: Sandwich-Bag Vegetables
Whole-wheat bread
Fruit

Dinner: Kasha (Buckwheat) and Fish
Steamed Vegetables
Orange

Day 10

Lunch: Rodeo and Wilshire Yogurt
Whole-wheat bread
1/2 melon or grapefruit

Dinner: Margarita's Black Beans and Rice
Crucifer and Carrot Slaw Salad
Banana and/or orange

Day 11

Lunch: Vegetable Soup
Pita Sandwich

Dinner: Chicken and Red Pepper Rice
Steamed Vegetables
Dr. Fox's Super Salad

Day
12

Lunch: Cold sliced chicken breast in pita
Fruit Salad

Dinner: Bean Lentil Supreme
Steamed Vegetables

Day
13

Lunch: Sandwich-Bag Vegetables
Crunchy Potato Salad
Apple

Dinner: Tuna Sprouts
Brown rice or barley
Shredded carrots and cabbage

Day
14

Lunch: Beverly Hills Coleslaw Salad
Tuna Sprouts in pita

Dinner: Mixed beans
Steamed Vegetables

How Much?

How much should you consume at each meal? It's best
to eat small portions of a variety of foods. Eat slowly;
when you eat rapidly your stomach fills up before your
brain gets the signal to turn off your appetite. Eat until
you feel almost full, then stop. A short time later your
brain will get the message, and you'll feel comfortable.

Never eat until you feel stuffed. The Super Food diet is more concerned with your "doctor within" and your immune system than with weight loss. If you wish to lose weight, eat more vegetables and less grains and beans.

Give It Time

The Super Food diet is based on something that many of us are unfamiliar with—the natural taste of food. We're so accustomed to fat, sugar and artificial flavors and textures we often turn up our noses at real, unadulterated food. I remember how hard it was, many years ago, to persuade my young children that apple juice was really brown in color, not yellowish.

Give your taste buds a little time to get used to food's natural flavors. At first you may miss the salt, gravies, sugar, sauces, oils and butter that we habitually pour all over our food. But soon you'll realize just how good fresh foods taste all by themselves.

Healthy Lunches at Work

Relatively few people consistently eat lunch at home. "How can I eat a decent lunch at the office?" many patients ask. Good, healthy lunches can be brought from home. Many of my patients who are executives, bankers, accountants and businesspeople carry their vegetables and other foods right in their briefcases. Bringing food to work is also less expensive than eating out all the time. Healthy and economical—what a deal! But if you must eat out, order lightly steamed vegetables, served without rich sauces or other foods prepared in the ways I have described.

Having mastered the Immune for Life philosophy of eating, and its daily applications, it's time to turn to the exercises that will benefit your "doctor within." In the next chapter you'll learn how brisk walking, as well as other exercises, help to make your "doctor within" as strong as it can be.

Chapter 4

Exercising Your "Doctor Within"

I was sitting in my office with a pleasant 42-year-old-banker. His medical and personal history had been taken, his physical examination was completed and his test results had been returned to me. His outlook on life was good, but his health was only fair. After discussing Super Foods and other recommendations, I suggested that he embark on a program of regular exercise. His reply went something like this:

"I'd like to, Dr. Fox, but I haven't got the time. Besides, I get enough exercise at work. I'm already in good shape, and I'm basically healthy, so I don't need to exercise. Plus, I eat well. That's not to say I wouldn't, but I really don't have the energy for exercise after a full day at work. And exercise would make me hungry; I'd eat more and get fat. You know, this exercise thing is just another fad like hoola hoops. Who runs a 10K anymore? What it comes down to is that exercise is boring. Besides, I'd be too embarrassed to work out at a club. Everybody there is in such good shape. I'd look like an overweight, out-of-shape old man."

This guy wins the best-excuse-for-not-exercising prize. But he loses the bigger prize: a chance to make his "doctor within" stronger and healthier.

The Average American:
Overweight and Out of Shape

An old friend from my Army days in Italy brought her family to visit mine some years ago. At the end of their stay she asked me why were so many Americans fat. And why do they drive around a parking lot six times looking for a parking space right next to the store? Why do they wait five minutes for an elevator rather than walk up one or two flights of stairs? "I think the only time they exercise," she said, "is when they run to the kitchen during television commercials."

She's right. The average American is overweight and out of shape. The average American would rather drive than walk three blocks to a store. And how many times have you been in an elevator and seen people ride up or down only one or two flights?

Like the 42-year-old-banker, most of us have many excuses for not exercising. My personal favorite is, "The dog looks too tired to go walking with me, so I won't take a walk." I've used this excuse myself plenty of times. That is, I used to.

An Inspiration

Then one day, while running in a 10K race at UCLA, I saw a paraplegic man, lying face down on a small, lightweight gurney, pulling himself along the course with two canes. He'd put one cane down and pull the gurney forward a few inches. Then he'd put the other cane down, pulling his gurney foward a few more inches. I wondered how he was going to make it up the hill, so I slowed down and trotted right behind him. He went right up that big hill, slowly, a few inches at a time. Drenched with sweat, huffing and puffing, he proudly finished the race, smiling at the applause he received as he struggled across the finish line.

If *he* can find the time, energy and discipline to exercise, I vowed, so can I. Since then, the dog has never looked too tired to go walking with me.

Do *you* set aside time for exercise? Have you the energy and discipline? In the Immune for Life Workbook, on page 200, you'll take a short quiz that will give you a close, hard look at your exercise attitudes and practices.

Why Exercise?

Let's begin with the psychological benefits. My experience with patients, confirmed by other studies, is that regular exercisers tend to have a more positive outlook on life. Regular exercise improves your health, and healthy people are generally happier people. People who exercise have the great satisfaction of knowing that they're working hard to strengthen their health; they have the discipline, energy and motivation to stick to their exercise program.

As we've seen, these positive feelings are mirrored by health-giving changes in body chemistry. Thus the pride, self-esteem and satisfaction that one derives from exercise goes a long way toward boosting one's "doctor within."

"I go out there and walk 30 minutes every day!" a patient will proudly announce. Or, "For the first time since I was a kid, I can easily touch my toes!" Some tell me that they can finally see their toes again now that they've lost a lot of weight. I've seen many poor self-images go way up as people prove to themselves that they can accomplish something worthwhile. This is especially true for the unhappy and depressed among us.

Unfortunately, millions of Americans are unhappy, with symptoms ranging from a simple indifference to enjoyment all the way to full-blown depression. Many studies have shown that one of the best, and simplest, treatments for depression is regular exercise.

Exercise and Endorphins

"You know, Dr. Fox," a formerly depressed, 22-year-old woman named Anne told me, "I stick to my exercise program. Even on days when I'm feeling lazy, I do it anyway. That means I've got more discipline and health-energy than more than half the people in the country. That makes me feel good."

When Anne said so emphatically that exercise improved her spirits, I began to wonder about the effect of exercise on her endorphins. I firmly believe that the positive feelings she got from exercising were raising her endorphins. As her good thoughts raised her endorphin levels, and otherwise improved her body chemistry, she couldn't help but feel better physically, mentally and emotionally.

Now let's look at just a few of the ways that exercise, combined with the rest of my Immune for Life program, can improve your physical health.

Exercice Strengthens Your Heart

Exercise has a very beneficial effect on your cardiovascular system (heart and blood circulation). The heart itself is a pumping muscle. Its ability to circulate blood and nutrients through your body depends on it being able to squeeze tightly over and over again, roughly 100,000 times a day. It's well known that the only way to strengthen a muscle and keep it strong is to use it. The more you use it the stronger it gets. Conversely, if you don't use it, you may lose it.

Regular, vigorous exercise makes your heart muscle stronger by giving it a good workout. There are some very good studies that compare heart attacks among regular exercisers and non- exercisers. Exercisers have stronger hearts than nonexercisers. If and when an exerciser has a heart attack, it will probably be less severe than the heart attack the nonexerciser suffers. The exerciser will also usually recover quicker.

Exercise Away Cholesterol

Exercise also helps to lower your cholesterol level, thus reducing your risk of heart disease. The cholesterol and fat-laden Standard American Diet encourages the formation of plugs in your arteries. It doesn't take much to completely block the tiny arteries that bring fresh blood to your heart muscle. That's why it's important to keep your cholesterol level low.

Regular exercise can lower your total cholesterol level, especially when combined with the Super Food diet. As the cholesterol level falls, so does your risk of having a heart attack. For every one-percent drop in your blood cholesterol, you'll enjoy a two-percent drop in your risk of developing coronary artery disease.

While lowering total cholesterol, exercise increases the levels of HDL (good) cholesterol. The risk of having a heart attack is inversely related to HDL: the higher your HDL, the lower the risk of heart disease. HDL has been compared to a garbage truck, taking cholesterol away from artery walls and down to the liver for disposal. (I like my patients to have HDLs of 50 or more.)

In addition, vigorous exercise lowers the LDL (bad) cholesterol. I've seen this happen frequently to my patients. LDL has been described as the "delivery truck" that brings cholesterol to the arteries, where it accumulates and narrows those vital passageways. You want to keep your LDL low, and exercise will help you do that.

Exercise Away Blood Fat

Exercise can also protect us against the dangers of excessive triglycerides. Triglycerides are the fats in your blood. Triglyceride levels rise when we eat foods containing fat. Ingesting alcohol and the refined carbohydrates found in cakes, pies, ice cream, candy, white-flour bread, pasta, etc., will also prompt a rise in your triglycerides. One of the problems with triglycerides is that they can help damage or plug arteries. If the triglycerides rise to very high levels, they can cause other diseases such as pancreatitis (inflammation of the pancreas). Pancreatitis may manifest itself as frequent episodes of upper abdominal pain. If it is severe enough it can lead to death.

We're all familiar with a very common problem associated with excess triglycerides: the fat that accumulates on us as our body stuffs triglycerides into fat cells. The only sensible way to get them out is by exercise and diet. With vigorous exercise, the triglycerides are pulled from the fat cells and broken down into free fatty acids, which the muscle cells can use for energy.

More serious, however, is the connection between fat and cancer. Everything you can do to keep your fat levels low—including exercise—is vitally important to avoid the killer cancers.

Exercise Lowers Blood Pressure

With continued exercise, the tiny blood vessels that carry fresh blood throughout your body begin to relax: resistance to the blood flow decreases, and blood pressure is lowered. This effect can last for many hours, during and after exercise. That's why it's especially important for people with high blood pressure to exercise.

> *NOTE: If you have high blood pressure or any other medical problems, see your doctor before beginning an exercise program.*

Exercise For Air

During exercise, your lungs work harder to make sure that enough oxygen gets into the blood. But it's the muscles between the ribs (intercostal muscles) and the diaphragm that actually tighten, then relax, to expand and contract your lungs. Like any other muscles, the intercostals and the diaphragm get stronger with use. In the long run, sustained exercise increases your ability to take oxygen into your lungs. I've found that pulmonary (lung) functions improve in almost all patients after just four to six weeks of regular exercise.

Tone Those Muscles

Muscles love to work; they were born to contract and relax and keep you moving. It's only with overuse or underuse that they have trouble. Put a trained athlete in bed for a week or so, and that person will lose up to 25 percent of his or her muscle strength. That's quite a lot.

Whether you're 30 or 70, you want your muscles to be well exercised and toned. Without good muscle tone we feel tired and weak and have difficulty at work, home and play. I use a dynamometer to measure the muscle strength in the hands of my patients. I find that people who can squeeze only 30 or 40 pounds of pressure can double or triple that figure after a simple exercise program. I'm not suggesting that you need to develop a bodybuilder's physique. Muscles do not need to be bulky, but they should be toned. Depending on the exercise, you can tone and stengthen various muscles in your body to give yourself a feeling of health and put a spring in your step.

Losing Weight Even When You're Not Exercising

One of the best ways to lose weight, and keep it off, is to exercise regularly and vigorously. Regular exercise gets the muscles working harder. The individual cells burn extra calories during exercise. And the cells continue to burn calories for hours, even after you've stopped exercising. That means you continue to lose weight even when you're not exercising.

Muscle cells use more energy at rest than fat cells do. So exercising, dieting away excess fat and building up weak muscles makes it easier for you to control your weight.

Exercise also helps control your appetite. Contrary to popular belief, vigorous exercise doesn't make you hungry. So regular exercise should be a part of any weight-control program—a lifelong program.

Exercise Equals Longevity

For the reasons I've just discussed, and more, exercise adds health and zest to your years, and years to your life. This has been confirmed by a long term study of 17,000 Harvard graduates. Those men who did enough exercise to burn at least 2,000 calories a week lived longer than those who exercised less or not at all. It takes the equivalent of about five hours of brisk walking, or four hours of jogging, to burn 2,000 calories.

Even the exercisers who had high blood pressure, a family history of early death or who smoked, benefited.

Walking Your "Doctor Within"

Caution: Check with your physician before beginning this or any other exercise program, and before making major changes in your exercise program.

The exercise program I recommend to my patients is very simple and easy to do. It requires no training or practice. There's nothing to learn, no special clothes or equipment to purchase, no clubs to join.

It begins with walking.

After carefully examining my patients to make sure they're able, I tell them to start by setting aside ten minutes every day for a brisk walk. How brisk? As brisk as you can make it: work up to double time.

The initial goal is ten consecutive minutes of brisk walking. How far you go isn't important. If ten minutes is too difficult at first, walk as much as you comfortably can, rest and then walk a little more at a slower pace.

When you can walk briskly for ten minutes without stopping, start increasing your time. Add two minutes to the ten, then another two and another two, and so on until you reach 25 minutes of nonstop, brisk walking. You've mastered brisk walking. You're giving your heart, lungs, legs and other parts of your body a real workout, and you're strengthening your "doctor within."

How long should it take to go from ten to 25 minutes? That depends on you. You're not training for the Olympics, and there are no deadlines. Yours is a program of lifelong exercise for the benefit of your "doctor within." Whether it takes two days or two months of practice to be able to walk 25 minutes nonstop is unimportant.

The Walking President

President Harry Truman had a regimen of brisk walking. He walked at the Army pace: 110 steps per minute. Reporters would often follow, throwing questions at him as they huffed and puffed along. They used to complain that he was walking too fast for them, even though they were younger than he was. When he came back to Washington for a visit he was in his 70's, the reporters had trouble keeping up with him.

The Formula for Success

Twenty five minutes of nonstop, brisk walking, four days a week, will boost your immune system, strengthen your heart and lungs, lower cholesterol levels, raise your HDL (good) cholesterol, tone your leg muscles, help control your weight and fight high blood pressure.

But 25 minutes a day, four days a week, isn't enough brisk walking to burn 2,000 calories a week. That's why it's very important to combine your regular brisk walking sessions with lots of spontaneous brisk walks to the store, around the neighborhood, up and down stairs, visiting your nearby friends and so on. Look for ways to add steps each day.

Walking Relieves Back Pain

Walking is actually good for your lower back. Standing up or walking is easier on your back than sitting down; the mechanical load is less. Most of my patients with lower-back pain report that regular walking helps relieve the pain. Furthermore, it helps reduce the distress and frustration caused by the pain.

Sometimes I have my lower-back-problem patients begin by walking slowly and gently, or walking only on soft, grassy surfaces. But soon, most of them are able and eager to walk briskly and get all the other benefits of this simple but very effective aerobic exercise.

Measuring Your Success

Use your heart to determine whether you're walking rapidly enough. Count your heartbeats by feeling your pulse at your wrist, your temples or on either side of your neck.

Count the number of times your heart beats in ten seconds. Multiply that number by six to get your heart rate per minute. The goal is to walk briskly enough to keep your heart beating at 70 to 80 percent of your maximal attainable heart rate. The 70 to 80 percent range will vary according to your age. Use the chart on page 117 to find your "Heartbeat Target Zone."

Check your pulse a couple of times during your walk, and again when you finish, to make sure you're pacing yourself just right.

Make Your Walking Fun

If you think daily walking would be boring, who says you have to walk by yourself? Years ago I took brisk evening strolls with my young children. We'd start from our house and walk all the way down the hill, then over to the shopping center. It was about a two-mile walk. Then I'd call my wife to bring the car and drive us back

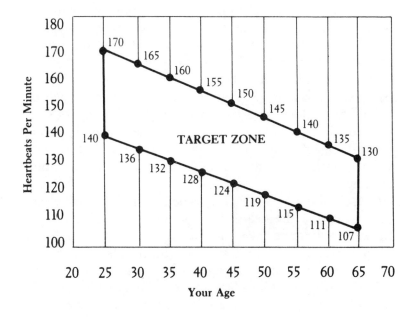

up the hill. (I would tell her the kids were too young to walk up the long, steep hill. The truth was I was too lazy.)

The time I spent walking with my children was great. We talked about baseball, medicine, history or whatever else was on our minds. They would tell me the latest jokes from school. Our walks were always enormous fun.

I've exercised with my family, friends, patients and business colleagues. While exercising I've chatted, conducted business, given medical advice, caught up with old friends and talked through ideas for books and articles with my son and coauthor, Barry.

And when I'm walking alone I use the time for sightseeing and mental relaxation. Sometimes I'll include streets such as Rodeo Drive in my exercise route. That gives me a chance to window-shop. Other times I'll walk in the park or among the beautiful houses of Beverly Hills. Walking is an exercise that leaves you free to think, see, hear, talk and laugh all you like.

Brisk walking, 25 minutes a day, four days a week, is enough to provide you with physical and psychological well-being. For the more eager and adventurous, there are many other great exercise activities.

Riding a bicycle is an excellent exercise, whether it be a real bicycle or an exercise bicycle. When it gets too hot or too cold to exercise outdoors, I go with my sons to a health club. While they're lifting weights and playing basketball, I ride a stationary bicycle and watch the pretty women lifting weights, stretching and taking aerobics classes.

Swimming is another excellent, all-around exercise that gives you the health benefits of brisk walking. And because swimming takes the weight off your lower back, it's a wonderful activity for those with problem backs.

Brisk walking, jogging, swimming, cross-country skiing, rowing, aerobics, karate—anything that keeps your heart beating in your Heartbeat Target Zone for about 25 minutes will do the trick. If you prefer more strenuous and difficult activities, fine. If not, brisk walking is all it takes to strengthen your "doctor within." Such sports as baseball and touch football are fun, but they don't give you the aerobic benefits of walking, because the action isn't continuous. Your heart rate doesn't stay in the Heartbeat Target Zone. Instead, it bounces up and down as you start and stop.

Wogging: The Happy Exercise

In one of my previous books, *The Beverly Hills Medical Diet*, I introduced an exercise I called wogging: a combination of walking and jogging. I explained how I wogged through Beverly Hills in the morning or evening, alternately walking one block and jogging one block, past the beautiful homes and shops.

Wogging is a happy exercise. I enjoy wogging around the high school track, where the regular joggers often stop me to enquire about my unique exercise. Other times you'll find me wogging through Beverly Hills. I wonder what the tourists on Rodeo Drive must think about the man they may have seen walking and jogging down that ritzy street?

Make sure to wear good-fitting, well-padded exercise shoes for wogging.

Exercises for the Belly

In addition to brisk walking, exercises that strengthen the back and stomach muscles are important. Seventy to 80 percent of adults have some form of lower back pain. Strengthening the back and stomach muscles helps prevent or alleviate the problem. People with chronic back pain are less likely to be physically active and more likely to be depressed. Getting rid of back pain allows you to be active again, and it helps get rid of or reduce depression. This, in turn, has a beneficial effect on your endorphins and health in general.

Here are three good exercises for the back and stomach. Take it easy in the beginning, adding repetitions as you go along. You'll find yourself becoming stronger and more energetic as you continue the exercise.

> *Caution: Do not do any of these exercises if you experience any pain while exercising. Stop and check with your physician before continuing your exercises. I don't believe that pain is necessary for gain.*

Shoulder Lifts: This exercise is good for your upper-abdominal and lower-back muscles. Lie on your back with your knees bent and feet flat on the floor. Clasp your hands behind your neck. Raise your shoulders up until they're several inches off the floor. Don't try to pull yourself up with your hands—use your abdominal muscles.

Do as many shoulder lifts as you can, even if it's only a few. Gradually work up to 50 shoulder lifts, twice a day. Then slowly work up to 100 shoulder lifts, twice a day.

Bicycle Riding: This is a good exercise for the lower-abdominal muscles. Lie on your back. Put your arms alongside your body, palms down. This helps steady your body. Bend your knees, then lift your thighs until they're at a 90-degree angle to your belly. Raise your legs so that they're parallel to the floor and in position to pedal an imaginary bicycle.

Pedal the imaginary bike, pumping your legs out (away from your body) and back in (toward your chest). Pedal as long as you can. Your initial goal is to be able to pedal the imaginary bicycle 100 times, times a day. Stay with it until you can pedal the imaginary bicycle 200 times without stopping.

Elbows to Knees: This is a good exercise for the upper- and lower-abdominal muscles, and it will help your back as well. Lie on your back. Clasp your hands behind your neck, elbows forward. Bend your knees, then lift them up and toward your chest, holding them over your belly. Your legs should be high in the air, with your toes pointing upward.

Raise your head and shoulders off the ground so that your elbows touch your knees. Lower your head and shoulders back to the ground, and repeat. Start by doing as many as you can, adding a few more every day. Your initial goal is 20 "elbows to knees," twice a day. Keep adding repetitions until you can easily do 100 without stopping.

It's a good idea to set goals for yourself as you progress through your exercise program. For example, decide that you're going to do 40 shoulder lifts today. If for any reason you can't do more than 20, well, do your 20, take a break and do the rest. That way, you have the pleasure of achieving your goal, even if you had to split the 40 in half.

By the way, one of my favorite approaches is to lie in front of the television set and watch the news as I ride my imaginary bicycle, do my shoulder lifts and elbows to knees. Or you can listen to music if you like.

Stretching

Due to our sedentary life-styles, we spend a great deal of time sitting down. This leads to the contraction of leg and back muscles. Stretching helps to prevent the muscles of the back and lower legs from becoming excessively tight. This, in turn helps to relieve the tension and pain that gathers in these muscles during the day. It's amazing how good you feel after your stretch out.

There are many good stretching books and programs available. You can stretch almost anywhere. In my office I stand about three feet from a wall, facing the wall. I lean up against the wall, the palms of my hands at about shoulder height, supporting my weight. Then I stretch my calf muscles (in the back of the lower legs) by pushing my heels toward the ground. I like to hold a comfortable (painless) stretch for three minutes, not bouncing back and forth, just holding the position. I also stretch my back muscles by bending over to touch my toes, although I can't quite reach my toes, and stay in this position for 20 or 30 seconds, several times a day. Finally, I stand with my feet about shoulder-width apart, arms half-way out at my sides, and turn from side to side, twisting at the hips to face to the right, then the left, over and over again, for 20 or 30 seconds. You don't have to be as flexible as a gymnast or a ballet dancer, but you should be able to twist, turn and move your muscles to meet the demands of everyday life. You'd be surprised at the number of my patients who have difficulty simply bending over to pick something up or turning their heads while driving to see if there's a car in the next lane! There's no medical problem making it so difficult for them to move; they've simply allowed their muscles to become very tight.

My general philosophy is to stretch whenever you can, which in my case means a few times a day. Again, stretch gently. If you're having pain, there's something wrong. Have your physician check it out. And always stretch before and after strenuous exercise.

Tone Your Muscles

As a rule, you can't feel good if your muscles are weak. Instead, you feel tired, below par. Feeling this way affects your emotional state. You probably feel depressed and unhappy with your inability to perform the activities you want to do. Many people tell me they can't carry bags of groceries because their arms feel too tired.

For these and other reasons, it's important that you tone the large-muscle groups in your arms and legs. Brisk walking or jogging tones your legs. Swimming tones arms and legs. For my arm exercise I keep two barbells near my bathroom sink. I turn on the Physician's Radio Network in the morning to hear the latest medical news while doing these three exercises for the muscles of my arms and shoulders. Start with light weights; three or five pounds is fine. I believe it's better to do more repetitions with light weights than to struggle through fewer repetitions with heavy weights. You can always increase the weight as you get stronger.

Bicep Curl: The biceps are the muscles on the "inside" of your upper arm, the muscles that tighten when somebody rolls up their sleeves and "makes a muscle." Hold one weight in each hand, with your arms resting at your sides. Your little fingers should be closest to your body, your thumbs furthest away. Keeping your elbows at your sides, lift your hands, bending your arms at the elbow, and bring the weights up until they almost touch the front of your shoulders. Then lower your arms back to the starting position and repeat. Do five to start. Gradually work up to 20 to 30 curls without stopping.

Shoulder press: This exercise is for the muscles of your upper arms and shoulders. Grasp a weight in each hand; lift and rest them on your shoulders. This is the starting position. Now, lift your hands straight up in the air, toward the ceiling. When your arms are extended fully above your shoulders, slowly bring them back to the starting position. Do this five to ten times, and gradually increase the repetitions as your muscles tone up. You should eventually be able to do 30 shoulder presses, twice a day.

Triceps Drop: This exercise is good for the tricep, which is the muscle on the back of the upper arm. I do one arm at a time. Holding a weight in my right hand, I lift my right arm straight into the air until it's locked in position above my shoulder. This is the starting position. Then, slowly bending my right elbow, I gently lower the weight behind my head, being careful not to hit myself in the head. When I feel the weight touching the base of my neck, I lift it back in the air until the arm is straight again. Start with five triceps drops, working up to 30 triceps drops with each arm, twice a day.

This is an important exercise, especially for women who complain of loose skin hanging from the back of their upper arms. If you keep the tricep muscles firm and filled out, there will be less likelihood of hanging skin.

You don't have to do these upper-body exercises exactly the way I do. If five-pound weights are too heavy for you, try three-pound, or one-pound weights. Or use books; they come in all sizes and weights. Cans are also useful weights. There are many good exercises for your arms and shoulders. Select the ones you like best, and make them part of your Immune for Life exercise program.

From Grumbler to Enthusiast

Mr. Green learned how beneficial walking can be when he flew in from Georgia for evaluation and treatment. He was suffering from heart trouble, weakness, fatigue, depression and general aches and pains. Since it would take about two weeks to give him a very thorough examination and design and implement a program for him, he and his wife checked into the Beverly Wilshire Hotel, a few blocks away from my office.

The first time he came to my office he leaned heavily on his cane, grumbling about having to "walk so far from the parking lot" next door. I examined him and determined that walking would be safe and beneficial. He laughed. "Walk? I can't walk from my bed to the bathroom!"

I put my foot down, figuratively speaking, and insisted that he walk from my office to the corner and back before he got in his car—a distance of about 50 yards. It took five minutes and a great deal of effort to cover the short distance, but he finally made it.

"I'll do it again tomorrow," he grumbled to me as he and his wife got into their rented car and drove off.

I don't know why he walked to the corner and back again the next day; he seemed to hate making the effort. But he did it, twice. The following day he insisted I join him for a walk around the block during lunch. "I practiced last night," he said with a grin. As we walked, I noticed he was leaning on his cane only lightly.

Mr. Green became quite enthusiastic about his walking. He wound up staying a full month at the Beverly Wilshire, coming to my office every day so I could monitor his progress and we could walk together. Soon he was taking four walks a day. As he shifted away from the Standard American Diet to one based on Super Foods, and continued to exercise, he began to feel increasingly better.

The Super Foods were very important, of course, but I think that exercise was the most important part of his treatment program; not because exercise is more important than diet, but because he was a businessman who liked to deal with things he could measure, and walking was a measureable and tangible achievement for him. Every day he told me proudly how many blocks he had walked the day before and what the running total was. By the end of the month he was able to walk 20 minutes without stopping, and without his cane. Before he left, he told me that learning that he could walk again had convinced him that he wasn't a helpless old man.

I hear from Mr. Green occasionally. He now walks briskly for 25 minutes every morning. "Just like the doctor ordered" he says.

Meditative Relaxation

Now that we've looked at the physical exercises that strengthen your "doctor within" let's examine a very different kind of exercise. You do these exercises sitting down, but they're just as important as all the others I've described.

I teach my patients a three-tiered program of Meditative Relaxation, designed to boost their "doctor within" and their immune system. The state of chronic stress so many of us live in depresses the immune system. These antistress techniques are designed to turn off the inappropriate production of those dangerous, high-voltage chemicals that are secreted during chronic stress.

Meditative Relaxation requires only 10 to 15 minutes, twice a day. Go into a room that has no telephone. Turn off the lights and close the curtains or shades. Tell everyone not to bother you.

Push a cozy chair up against a wall, and sit comfortably in that chair. Plant your feet squarely on the floor, just a bit in front of you. If you can feel your belt, tie or other tight clothing, loosen or unbutton the offending article. Put your hands on your knees, and you're ready to begin.

I suggest you get the feel of the exercise by reading through the entire three-part program several times, out loud. If you desire, read the whole program into a tape recorder, and play it back when you're ready for your Meditative Relaxation sessions.

Part One: Tensing for Relaxation

Begin by tensing and relaxing your eyes, mouth, neck, arms, trunk and legs. To help my patients remember the sequence, I write this sentence on a card and give it to them: Every Muscle Needs A Total Loosening.

Every = eyes	A = arms
Muscle = mouth	Total = trunk
Needs = neck	Loosening = legs

Every Muscle Needs A Total Loosening: Memorize this sentence.

Every = Eyes

Begin by closing your eyes. Hold them clenched shut, as tightly as you can. Clench them still tighter. Hold the muscles taut while you count: one thousand ... two thousand ... three thousand ... four thousand ... five thousand ... six thousand ... seven thousand ... eight thousand ... nine thousand ... ten thousand. Count slowly.

Relax your eye muscles.

Now take a slow, deep breath in through your nose. Hold it. Then let it slowly out through your mouth, very slowly, taking at least five seconds to let it all out.

Take another slow breath. Fill your lungs. Feel your diaphragm pulling down to open the lungs wide. With your mind's eye, see your diaphragm dropping down as your lungs fill.

Now repeat. Squeeze your eyes tightly shut. Hold your eyes closed tightly while you count, slowly: one thousand ... two thousand ... three thousand ... four thousand ... five thousand ... six thousand ... seven thousand ... eight thousand ... nine thousand ... ten thousand.

Slowly relax your muscles, and slowly open your eyes.

Take a deep breath in through your nose ... a nice, deep breath. Feel your diaphragm pulling down to open your lungs wide. In your mind's eye, see your diaphragm dropping down as your lungs fill.

Hold the breath for a moment. Now let it out through your mouth, very slowly, taking at least five seconds to empty your lungs.

Take another big breath, and fill up your lungs.

Hold it for a moment. Now let it out very slowly. Take five seconds or more to blow it all out.

The muscles around your eyes don't feel tired anymore. They feel good.

Muscle = Mouth

Now tighten up the muscles of your mouth. Grimace. Show your teeth, and tighten up the muscles around your mouth and the front of your neck. Tilt your chin up. Now, with your teeth still bared, open your lips as wide as you can. Hold them open, teeth clenched, as you also tighten your cheek and neck muscles. Teeth clenched, cheeks and neck tight, lips pulled open, hold these muscles tight while you count: one thousand ... two thousand ... three thousand ... four thousand ... five thousand ... six thousand ... seven thousand ... eight thousand ... nine thousand ... ten thousand. Count slowly.

Slowly relax your lips, jaw, cheek and neck muscles.

Take in a deep breath through your nose, filling your lungs as you feel your diaphragm pulling down to open your lungs and make room for the air.

Hold the breath for a moment. Now let it go very slowly, taking at least five seconds to let it all out.

Take another breath. Fill your lungs. Feel your diaphragm pulling down to open your lungs wide. With your mind's eye, see your diaphragm dropping down as your lungs fill.

Now repeat. Tighten the muscles of your mouth, clench your teeth and grimace. Tilt your chin up and tighten the muscles around your mouth and in the front of your neck. Hold that for a moment, then open your lips as wide as you tighten your cheek and neck muscles. Hold those muscles tight while you count, slowly: one thousand ... two thousand ... three thousand ... four thousand ... five thousand ... six thousand ... seven thousand ... eight thousand ... nine thousand ... ten thousand.

Slowly relax your jaw, lips, cheek and neck muscles.

Take a deep breath in through your nose ... a nice, deep breath. Feel your diaphragm pulling down to open your lungs wide. See, in your mind's eye, your diaphragm dropping down as your lungs fill.

Hold the breath for a moment. Now let it out through your mouth very slowly, taking at least five seconds to empty your lungs.

Take another deep breath, filling up your lungs.

Hold it for a moment. Now let it out, very slowly. Take five seconds or more to blow it all out.

The muscles of your mouth and the front of your neck now feel light and relaxed.

Needs = Neck

Next comes the neck. Gently but firmly push your head against the wall behind you. This puts the muscles in the back of your neck into a contraction. Hold that position while you count: one thousand ... two thousand ... three thousand ... four thousand ... five thousand ... six thousand ... seven thousand ... eight thousand ... nine thousand ... ten thousand. Count slowly.

Slowly relax, letting your head slump forward just a little.

Take a deep breath in through your nose and hold it for a moment. Now blow it out through your mouth, very slowly, taking at least five seconds to let it all out.

Take another breath ... hold it ... let it out slowly.

Again. Gently but firmly push your head against the wall behind you. Hold that position while you count: one thousand ... two thousand ... three thousand ... four thousand ... five thousand ... six thousand ... seven thousand ... eight thousand ... nine thousand ... ten thousand. Count slowly.

Slowly relax, letting your head slump forward just a little.

Take a deep breath in through your nose and hold it for a moment. Now blow it out through your mouth, very slowly, taking at least five seconds to let it all out.

Take another breath ... hold it ... let it out slowly.

Now push up your shoulders so that they almost touch your ears. Tilt your chin up and your head back, so that the back of your head almost touches your raised shoulders. Push your neck down and back, into your shoulders, feeling the muscles at the base of your neck, where your neck meets your shoulders, contracting. Lift your shoulders up into your neck as high as you can. Feel the tension in the back of your neck and upper shoulders as you count slowly: one thousand ... two thousand ... three thousand ... four thousand ... five thousand ... six thousand ... seven thousand ... eight thousand ... nine thousand ... ten thousand.

Slowly relax your neck and lower your shoulders.

Take a deep breath in through your nose ... a nice deep breath. Hold the breath for a moment. Now let it out slowly, very slowly, through your mouth, taking at least five seconds to let it all out.

Take another deep breath, filling up your lungs.

Hold it for a moment. Now let it out, very slowly. Take five seconds or more to blow it all out.

Once more, tilt your neck back, and lift your shoulders up into your neck. Hold your neck and shoulders tense as you count slowly: one thousand ... two thousand ... three thousand ... four thousand ... five thousand ... six thousand ... seven thousand ... eight thousand ... nine thousand ... ten thousand.

Relax your neck and slowly lower your shoulders.

Take a deep breath in through your nose ... hold it ... let it out through your mouth, slowly, taking at least five seconds to let it all out.

Another deep breath ... hold it ... let it out slowly.

The muscles of your shoulders and the back of your neck now feel light and tingly.

A = Arms

Put both arms straight out in front of you at about shoulder height, palms facing down. Make two very tight fists, as tight as you can make them. Bending at the wrist, push your fists down toward the floor as hard as you can. Feel the muscles in your wrists and forearms tighten, and feel the tension, especially in your forearms, up to your elbows. Hold that position and count: one thousand ... two thousand ... three thousand ... four thousand ... five thousand ... six thousand ... seven thousand ... eight thousand ... nine thousand ... ten thousand.

Slowly relax. Open your fists. Rest your hands, palms down, on your knees. Feel how relaxed, refreshed and tingly your hands, wrists and arms feel.

Now, take in a deep breath through your nose. Hold it for a moment. Let it out very slowly, through your mouth, taking at least five seconds to let it all out.

Take another breath ... hold it ... let it out slowly.

Again. Put both arms straight out in front of you at about shoulder height, palms facing down. Make two very tight fists, as tight as you can make them. Bending at the wrist, push your fists down toward the floor as hard as you can. Feel the muscles in your wrists and forearms tighten, and feel the tension, especially in your forearms, up to your elbows. Hold that position and count: one thousand ... two thousand ... three thousand ... four thousand ... five thousand ... six thousand ... seven thousand ... eight thousand ... nine thousand ... ten thousand.

Slowly relax. Open your fists. Rest your hands, palms down, on your knees. Feel how relaxed, refreshed and tingly your hands, wrists and arms feel.

Now, take in a deep breath through your nose. Hold it for a moment. Let it out very slowly, through your mouth, taking at least five seconds to let it all out.

Take another breath ... hold it ... let it out slowly.

Now hold your arms out to the sides of your body at shoulder level, palms up. Close your hands into tightly clenched fists. Bend your arms at the elbow, bringing your fists to your ears. Clench your arm and shoulder muscles, especially the bicep muscles in your upper arms. Hold tight and count: one thousand ... two thousand ... three thousand ... four thousand ... five thousand ... six thousand ... seven thousand ... eight thousand ... nine thousand ... ten thousand.

Slowly relax, dropping your arms to your lap as you take in a deep breath through your nose.

Take in a deep breath through your nose. Hold it for a moment. Now, let it out slowly, very slowly, through your mouth, taking at least five seconds to empty your lungs.

Take another big breath, filling up your lungs.

Hold it for a moment. Now, let it out slowly, very slowly.

Again. Hold your arms out to the sides of your body at shoulder level, palms up. Close your hands into tightly clenched fists. Bend your arms at the elbow, bringing your fists to your ears. Clench your arm and shoulder muscles, especially the bicep muscles in your upper arms. Hold tight and count: one thousand ... two thousand ... three thousand ... four thousand ... five thousand ... six thousand ... seven thousand ... eight thousand ... nine thousand ... ten thousand.

Slowly relax, dropping your arms to your lap as you take in a deep breath through your nose.

Take in a deep breath through your nose. Hold it for a moment. Now let it out slowly, very slowly, through your mouth, taking at least five seconds to empty your lungs.

Take another big breath, filling up your lungs.

Hold it for a moment. Now, let it out, slowly, very slowly. For just a moment, concentrate on your arms. Feel how light and tingly they are.

Total = Trunk

Fill your lungs with as much air as you can. Holding the air in your lungs, bear down as if you were going to have a bowel movement. While holding the air and bearing down, place your fists up by your chin. Squeeze your arms tightly against your chest. Feel the tension in your chest muscles as you slowly count: one thousand ... two thousand ... three thousand ... four thousand ... five thousand ... six thousand ... seven thousand ... eight thousand ... nine thousand ... ten thousand.

Slowly relax, letting the air out of your lungs.

Now, take in a deep breath through your nose. Hold it for a moment. Let it slowly out through your mouth, very slowly, taking at least five seconds to let it all out.

Take another breath ... hold it ... let it out slowly.

Fill your lungs once again, bear down, hold your fists by your chin and squeeze your arms against your chest. Hold that position, chest muscles clenched tightly, as you count slowly: one thousand ... two thousand ... three thousand ... four thousand ... five thousand ... six thousand ... seven thousand ... eight thousand ... nine thousand ... ten thousand.

Slowly relax and exhale.

Take in a deep breath through your nose ... a nice, deep breath.

Hold the breath for a moment. Now let it out slowly, very slowly, through your mouth, taking at least five seconds to empty your lungs.

Take another big breath, filling up your lungs.

Hold it for a moment. Now let it out very slowly.

Your trunk now feels relaxed.

Loosening = Legs

Straighten out your legs in front of you, lock your knees and raise your feet off the floor. Hold them at about the level of your chair seat, toes pointing forward. Feel the tension in your calves, ankles, and in the front and outside of your thighs. Hold that position. Keep your toes pointed forward as you slowly count: one thousand ... two thousand ... three thousand ... four thousand ... five thousand ... six thousand ... seven thousand ... eight thousand ... nine thousand ... ten thousand.

Slowly relax, lowering your feet to the floor.

Now take in a deep breath through your nose. Hold it for a moment. Let it out through your mouth, very slowly, taking at least five seconds to let it all out.

Take another breath ... hold it ... let it out slowly.

Again, lift your feet off the floor, knees locked, toes pointing forward. Hold tight and count: one thousand ...

two thousand ... three thousand ... four thousand ... five thousand ... six thousand ... seven thousand ... eight thousand ... nine thousand ... ten thousand.

Slowly relax and exhale.

Take in a deep breath through your nose ... a nice, deep breath.

Hold the breath for a moment. Now let it out through your mouth, very slowly, taking at least five seconds to empty your lungs.

Take another big breath, and fill up your lungs.

Hold it for a moment. Now let it out very slowly.

Your leg muscles feel relaxed. It feels good.

You've relaxed your whole body. Now go back to the neck and shoulders one more time. Push the neck down and slightly back. Raise your shoulders up into your neck. Hold them tight as you count: one thousand ... two thousand ... three thousand ... four thousand ... five thousand ... six thousand ... seven thousand ... eight thousand ... nine thousand ... ten thousand.

Relax and take a deep breath. Hold it, then exhale slowly, taking at least five seconds to let it all out.

Another breath ... hold it ... let it out slowly.

Push your neck back down and your shoulders up one more time. Clench those muscles and count: one thousand ... two thousand ... three thousand ... four thousand ... five thousand ... six thousand ... seven thousand ... eight thousand ... nine thousand ... ten thousand.

The muscles in your neck feel relaxed.

Part Two: Concentration on Relaxation

Now your entire body is nice and relaxed. Get comfortable in your chair, keeping your feet on the floor. Close your eyes. You're going to become aware of various parts of your body. You're going to actually "feel" them. Breathe in and out slowly through your nose, concentrating on your feet. Relax and focus on your feet. See your feet with your mind's eye ... both of your feet ... toes ...

along your soles from your toes to your heels ... along the top from toes to the ankles. Feel your feet relaxing. Feel all of your toes relaxing ... your right and left soles ... right and left heels ... the tops of both your feet relaxing. Silently tell yourself that both feet are totally relaxed ... your toes, soles, heels, tops and bottoms of both your feet are totally relaxed.

Now feel your ankles relaxing. Concentrate on both your left and right ankle as you continue breathing through your nose, in and out, slowly. Feel both ankles. See them, in your mind's eye, relaxing. Silently tell yourself that your ankles are relaxed.

Continue breathing in and out through your nose, slowly, as you feel relaxation spreading to your calves, on the back sides of your lower legs. See them with your mind's eye. Concentrate on the feeling as both of your calves relax. Silently tell yourself that your calves are now relaxed.

With your calves relaxed, the feeling spreads around the front of your legs to your shins. Feel your right and left shins relaxing. See your shins with your mind's eye; feel them relaxing. Silently tell yourself that your shins are relaxed.

Continue breathing slowly through your nose, eyes closed, as you feel your knees relaxing. Concentrate on your left and right knees as you tell yourself that they are relaxed. See your knees with your mind's eye. Silently tell yourself that both of your knees are now relaxed.

Eyes closed, continue to breathe slowly, in and out through your nose, as you concentrate on your upper legs. See your upper legs, left and right, in your mind's eye. Feel the front of your upper legs relaxing. Now the relaxed feeling begins to spread to the outsides of your thighs ... to the bottoms of both your thighs. Concentrate on your upper legs as the relaxation moves back up the insides ... around to the tops. Silently tell yourself that both of your legs, from toes to thighs, are totally relaxed. And so they are.

As you continue breathing slowly through your nose

... slowly ... eyes closed ... feel your buttocks and genital area relaxing. Concentrate on the feeling of relaxing. Silently tell yourself that these areas are relaxed.

Continue concentrating as the relaxed feeling spreads to your lower abdomen, below your navel. Concentrate as the feeling of relaxation spreads through your lower abdomen. Eyes closed, breathing slowly through your nose, feel the relaxation. Silently tell yourself that your lower abdomen is relaxed.

Now feel your lower back relaxing, loosening up. Concentrate on the feeling of relaxation in your lower back. See your lower back in your mind's eye. Silently tell yourself that your lower back is relaxed. Feel the tension gathered in your lower back fading away.

Move your mind's eye up a little to focus on your belly, from your navel to your chest. Feel the relaxation moving up past your navel to your lower chest. Concentrate on the feeling of relaxation. Silently tell yourself that you're relaxed from your navel to your chest.

Now the relaxed feeling continues up your chest to the base of your neck. See your chest with your mind's eye. Focus on the pleasant feeling of relaxation as it covers your entire chest. Silently tell yourself that your chest is now relaxed.

Eyes still closed, breathing slowly ... in and out through your nose ... concentrate on the relaxation as it spreads over your upper back. See your upper back with your mind's eye. Concentrate on the relaxation as it covers your entire upper back. Silently tell yourself that your back, belly and chest are now totally relaxed.

Concentrate as the great feeling of relaxation continues up into your shoulders. See your shoulders ... left and right ... in your mind's eye. Feel the tension and tightness drain from both shoulders. Eyes closed, breathing slowly in and out through your nose, concentrate as your shoulders totally relax. Silently tell yourself that your shoulders are now relaxed.

Now the feeling of relaxation spreads up through your neck, from the bottom to the top. See your neck with your mind's eye. Feel the front of your neck relax. Concentrate as the feeling spreads around the right side of your neck ... the back ... the left side. Silently tell yourself that your whole neck is now completely relaxed.

Eyes closed, slowly breathing in and out through your nose, concentrate on the feeling of relaxation as it moves from your shoulders down both your arms. Picture your arms in your mind's eye. From your shoulders, the feeling of relaxation moves into the left and right upper arms ... front and back ... to both elbows ... front and back ... to your forearms ... front and back. Concentrate on the relaxation as it envelops both of your arms. Now your wrists are relaxing ... both wrists are relaxing. Concentrate as your fingers relax ... the fingers on both hands ... your thumbs ... index fingers ... middle fingers ... ring fingers ... little fingers. Silently tell yourself that both of your arms ... from your shoulders to the tips of each finger ... are relaxed.

Eyes closed, breathing slowly through your nose, see your head in your mind's eye. Concentrate on your head as the relaxation spreads up from your neck to your chin ... from the sides of your neck to the sides of your head ... from the back of your neck up the back of your head. Feel the relaxation spreading over your head ... your cheeks ... mouth ... nose ... eyes ... temples ... ears ... forehead. Concentrate carefully as the relaxation spreads up your head to the very top. Silently tell yourself that your head is now relaxed.

With your whole body totally relaxed, focus on your left arm. Eyes closed, breathing slowly through your nose, silently tell yourself that your left arm is heavy, very heavy. Feel your left arm becoming heavy. See it in your mind's eye, heavy. Concentrate on the feeling of heaviness.

Now see your right arm in your mind's eye. Concentrate on your right arm ... silently tell yourself that your right arm is heavy, very heavy. Feel your right arm becoming heavy. Concentrate on the feeling of heaviness in your right arm.

Now let the heaviness totally drain out of both arms.

Your breathing is slow and easy; your whole body is relaxed.

Part Three: "One"

As soon as you've completed your relaxation exercise, move right into meditation. You're totally relaxed. Keep your eyes closed. Silently, to yourself, begin saying "one" over and over again. Say it slowly. If you can sense your heartbeat, say "one" in time with your heart. If not, say it slowly, over and over again.

Now see the numeral "1" with your mind's eye. See it and say it silently, slowly, over and over. Don't count the number of times you say "one." Just keep seeing and saying it. If you get tired of the number "1," switch over to the word "one." See the three letters, "o," "n" and "e" with your mind's eye.

If your mind begins to wander, if you start thinking about work or supper, gently bring your attention back to "one."

If you can, see the "one" in color. See it in soft blue, with your mind's eye. See it in green, the green of trees in the woods. (When you can see it in color, or against a background, you know you're doing something powerful with your mind.)

Keep seeing and saying "one" until you feel it's time to stop. Don't set an alarm to go off at a certain time. You'll know when the session should end. Ten or fifteen minutes for the entire relaxation-meditation session should be enough, but no more than 20 minutes.

When you're finished, slowly open your eyes. Sit quietly for a few moments, then rise and go about your business.

Meditative Relaxation for Arthritis

I've found Meditative Relaxation to be especially helpful for my arthritic patients. I have them spend extra time relaxing their painful and/or swollen joints. A person with arthritis in the knuckles and fingers of the right hand, for example, adds this to the second part of the Meditative Relaxation: eyes closed, breathing slowly through your nose, picture your right hand with your mind's eye. Focus on the five knuckles ... and the thumb and fingers ... of your right hand. Now, with your mind's eye, see your right little finger. See your little finger and little-finger knuckle. Concentrate on your little finger and knuckle as the feeling of relaxation enters the knuckle ... spreads up through your finger ... from your knuckle ... through your little finger ... front, back and sides ... to the tip of your little finger. Now, with your mind's eye, see your right ring finger and ring-finger knuckle. Concentrate on your ring finger and knuckle as the soothing feeling of relaxation enters your ring-finger knuckle. From the knuckle the relaxation moves up to your ring finger ... all the way up your ring finger ... front, back and sides ... to the tip. Now, with your mind's eye, see your right middle finger and middle-finger knuckle. Concentrate on your middle finger and middle-finger knuckle. Concentrate as you feel the cooling, soothing relaxation enter your middle-finger knuckle. From the knuckle the relaxation moves slowly up your middle finger ... from your knuckle ... through your middle finger ... front, back and sides ... all the way to the tip of your finger. Next is your index finger and index-finger knuckle. See your index finger and index-finger knuckle with your mind's eye. Concentrate on your index finger and knuckle as the great feeling of relaxation and loosening enters the knuckle. From the knuckle it slowly spreads to your index finger ... up your finger ... front, back and sides ... all the way up your finger to the tip. Now concentrate on your right thumb and thumb knuckle. Focus on your right thumb and thumb knuckle. Feel the relief as the relaxation moves into the knuckle ... from your knuckle into your thumb ... up the thumb ... front, back and sides ... all the way up your thumb to the tip.

See your entire right hand with your mind's eyes. Hold that picture in your mind. Feel how relaxed your fingers and knuckles are. Keep your mind focused on that great feeling. Silently tell yourself that the fingers and knuckles on your right hand are relaxed.

Meditative Relaxation can be adapted to suit your specific needs. Do the complete session for the entire body, then adapt Part Two, as I've just done, to cover your special problem areas. You can focus in on muscles, joints or any part of your body you desire. One of my patients, an office worker, spends extra time relaxing her neck, shoulders, upper and lower back. These are the muscles that tighten up and hurt when she becomes stressed at work.

Using Meditative Relaxation

I suggest that you use Meditative Relaxation twice a day. Middle or late morning and late afternoon are good times. If you find yourself feeling run down in the early afternoon, do the Meditative Relaxation exercise during your lunch or coffee break.

I caution against doing it late at night. Why? Because you may feel too good to go to sleep.

Exercising Your "Doctor Within"

I urge all my patients to give their "doctor within" a good workout by walking briskly and enthusiastically, then sitting down to practice these relaxation exercises as well. For a small investment of time, you can immeasureably strengthen and energize your entire immune system.

Don't forget to take the exercise quiz in the Immune for Life Workbook on page 200. It will help you assess your exercise attitudes and practices and will be used in selecting the Nutri-Prevention supplement program you should consider in Part Two.

Chapter 5

Melding Mind and Body

A young woman sat in my office and said, "Whatever I do turns out wrong. I've been on five or six diets, but I can't lose any weight. I've gone to three colleges in seven years, and I'll never graduate. All I can get are jobs as a clerk or waitress. Then I do a lousy job and get fired after a while. I make resolutions to study harder, to work harder, to get along with my boyfriend. Nothing ever goes right for me! I don't even try anymore because I know I'm a loser." Like millions of Americans, she is depressed and has a negative self-image. She "knows" she's a loser. Her conviction becomes a self-fulfilling prophecy as she fails at one thing after another.

These unhappy people often wind up in doctors' offices, complaining of various aches and pains, if they're lucky. The unlucky ones may have more serious problems, such as cancer. These people aren't hypochondriacs suffering from imaginary diseases. Depression and unhappiness cause real physical illnesses.

Other patients I see are angry, eager to take on the whole world, to get back at someone, to show everybody

141

what's what. Herb A. was like that; he couldn't wait to make his old boss eat his words.

"Dr. Fox, I'm going to make him so sorry he fired me!" Herb fumed. "He said I didn't run my department the right way. Well, I'm going to get a job with a bigger firm, take over the whole company and run it my way. That'll show him! I'm going to buy him out, too. Just so I can fire him!"

The only person Herb showed was himself. His constant state of anger drove his blood pressure higher and higher until he had a heart attack.

Unfortunately, these people aren't alone in their gloomy thoughts. Tens of millions of Americans are depressed, angry, bitter and frustrated. Many of them turn to alcohol, tranquilizers and other prescription or illegal drugs. Thanks to the magic of chemistry, they lose themselves for a little while. But the real problems haven't been solved; the depression, anger and self-doubt always return. Meanwhile, the drugs and alcohol are busy attacking their body, destroying their relationships, harming their ability to work, draining their bank accounts and deepening their anger and/or depression.

Many of the patients I've seen through the years have told me that they can't get through the day without a tranquilizer, a few drinks or some marijuana. When I ask them if the drugs and/or alcohol make them any happier, they shrug and say no, but at least they're surviving. My goal for you isn't merely survival; it's living life to its fullest. Dimming the lights of thought and perception isn't living.

The Factory of the Mind

Your thoughts are the key. Thoughts become beliefs; thoughts and beliefs together help determine whether "good" or "bad" messages are sent from your brain to the rest of your body, including your immune system. What you think can literally make you sick or healthy.

Your mind is like a factory, filled with assembly lines producing chemical messages. Speeding along the various pathways in your body, the messages bring happiness, depression, health or disease. How do you know what the message will be? You create many of the messages with your thoughts. You, and only you, determine if they are messages of joy or despair.

What are some of the "bad" messages? Anger and rage result in the production of large amounts of epinephrine (adrenaline) and other powerful chemicals. Long-term manufacture and release of these strong substances can lead to elevated blood pressure, heart disease, ulcers and other problems. Depression and self-doubt spur the synthesis of hormones such as cortisone. Cortisone is an important and necessary body substance, but too much of it can have a deadly effect on your immune system, encouraging infections and even cancer.

The messages you want to see spread through your body are those of health and happiness. And for that you must look to hormones such as the endorphins. As Barry and I explained in our book, *DLPA to End Chronic Pain and Depression* (1985), the endorphins, produced by various cells in your body, are responsible for lifting your mood and blocking certain kinds of pain. It's postulated that chronic pain and depression are related to a deficiency of endorphins in the body.

Endorphins and the Immune System

Endorphins aren't satisfied with merely relieving pain and lifting your mood, however. They also work with your immune system to fight off disease. Certain immune-system cells have receptors that allow them to "communicate" with endorphins. Studies have shown that elevating endorphin levels can make the immune system operate more effectively. Endorphins enhance the "fighting" activity of some of your immune-system cells and help others chase after harmful substances in the body.

Think Endorphins: Think Love

Since endorphins lift our mood, quell pain and work hand-in-hand with our immune system, what can we do to make sure our endorphin levels are every bit as high as they should be? One way to keep the endorphins flowing is to be in love with someone, some thing, an idea or a cause.

What happens when you're at a party and you see an intriguing person across the room? Messages flash through your brain, and pretty soon you're standing next to him or her smiling and talking. If the "chemistry" is right, you may notice a tight feeling in your stomach and a flushed, warm sensation in your face and neck. You may not realize that your eyes are dilated, but you can feel your heart pounding and perspiration gathering on your body. As the romance builds and continues, you find that just being with him or her makes you feel great. Is it your loved one who "makes" you feel so good? No. It's you: your own reactions to that person.

Love beautifully illustrates the power of the mind. Decide that someone is the one for you, and a carefully orchestrated series of changes occur in your body. Chemicals scurry about your body, keeping your energy levels and enthusiasm sky high.

Like any happy, positive feeling, being in love increases the levels of substances such as endorphins, which not only make you feel great but strengthen your immune system as well. What a great way to fight disease!

The actual series of events in your brain and body is complex, but it boils down to the thoughts you think having a direct effect on your "doctor within" and your health. Love can be among the strongest of positive thoughts, so always look for ways to increase your openness to, and capacity for, love.

Thoughts Can Raise Endorphins

Love, of course, isn't the only good feeling that will increase endorphins. Let me tell you about a study conducted at the University of Tennessee a few years ago. The endorphin levels in the spinal fluid of 32 chronic-pain sufferers were measured; then the participants were given a placebo.

Placebos aren't medicine; they're "sugar pills." Surprisingly, they work just like real medicine for about one third of patients. In this study, the 14 patients who responded to the placebo were retested: their endorphin levels had increased!

It wasn't the placebo that made their endorphin levels rise; it was their *belief*. They thought the placebo was real medicine, so they believed it would relieve their pain. They felt so good about it that their bodies started producing extra endorphins, which blocked the pain. From belief to relief: it's a magical, but very real, process you can learn to use yourself.

Unfortunately, most of us mass-produce unhappy, unhealthy messages, flooding our bodies with chemical doomsayers. The tens of millions of Americans who are unhappy, depressed, angry, bitter, frustrated, feel inadequate, unloved, helpless and hopeless turn negative feelings into negative hormones into disease. That's the other side of the coin, the one we want to avoid.

Where Do Our Thoughts Come From?

"I'd like to think nice thoughts and have lots of endorphins, Dr. Fox," some of my patients say, "but everyone keeps making me mad. It's not my fault. It's my boss, my kids, the traffic, the economy. It's all those things that make me mad."

"We've been taught that our thoughts come from outside of us: someone or something imposes them on us. For example, we say: "He makes me so mad!" as if "I" have nothing to do with it; "I" am an innocent bystander.

"He" doesn't make you angry, calm, happy, or sad. "He" does nothing but provide a stimulus, some data for your brain. You make yourself angry, or calm, or happy, or sad by reacting to the stimulus.

Facts are Facts, Not Emotions

When your mind receives a piece of information, it responds by sending a chemical message to the appropriate part of your body. For example, when your eyes see that the traffic light is turning red, the brain interprets that fact and sends a "hit the brake" message to your right foot.

The red light was only a fact. It didn't "make" you step on the brake. It was your interpretation of the red light, combined with the knowledge that you were driving a car, and the light was so far away, and you were going so fast, etc., that persuaded you to brake. The red light was only one fact among many.

Remember that time, late at night, when you walked down a dark street in a not-so-nice part of town? As you looked into the shadows, and turned your head to see if anyone was behind you, your heart began to pound. You could feel your breath coming in short gasps as your muscles tensed and you began to sweat. Chemical fireworks were exploding inside of you, dilating your pupils for better vision, shutting down temporarily unnecessary actions like digestion, and rushing blood to your muscles, for example, to help you fight or run.

It took only a split second to turn you from a calm stroller into a frightened, highly charged person, ready to fight or run for his or her life. And what triggered this "fight or flight" response? Nothing but your thoughts. Nobody pulled a gun on you; nobody mugged you, nobody shouted at you or ran after you or made a threatening gesture. As a matter of fact, you never saw or heard anybody at all, because the street was deserted. You turned on the chemical fireworks with your thoughts.

You're in the Driver's Seat

You are the only one thinking in your head. You, and only you, determine what your thoughts will be. You control your interpretation of the facts coming into your mind. Your interpretation, in turn, determines your thoughts and your response.

You can't always decide which facts your brain will be receiving, but you have absolute control over your response. You decide how to interpret your world. You decide to get angry, to rage and fume and raise your blood pressure. You decide to be unhappy, to doubt yourself. You're in the driver's seat.

I don't mean to say, of course, that you should never be angry or unhappy. Sometimes these are very appropriate responses. If you're being cheated, or even mugged, some anger might help you fight back. When a loved one dies, of course you're unhappy. That's only natural. The problem lies in excess; too much anger or unhappiness produces too many of the harmful chemicals that ride roughshod over your "doctor within."

And not all of our thoughts are generated strictly by outside events. Many come from the good and bad memories we replay, like old movies, in the theater of our mind. Memories can stimulate very intense feelings. Don't you feel good when your mother tells a funny story from your childhood? Or when you remember how you hit the home run in Little League that won the game? What about how bad you feel when you rehash the memory of being turned down for a date?

You've got lots of old memory movies to play and replay. So stick with the oldies but goodies, and the new ones showing you as you *want* yourself to be. Leave those bad memories buried in the vault.

Is Stress Good or Bad?

Anger, rage, bitterness, depression, self-doubt, feelings of helplessness and so on, are all negative forms of stress. Stress is the response of your body, mind, emotions or spirit to any demand made upon them. Your life is constantly changing and may be stressful because all of these elements have to continually adapt to new demands made upon them. Some stress is necessary and good.

Cheering when your favorite team scores points is exciting and stressful, but it's good stress. Good stress has been called the spice of life. Without good stress, life would be deadly boring.

The stress I experienced when I first kissed my wife-to-be over 30 years ago was good stress. It must have been—I immediately fell down the steps. (Talk about a powerful kiss!) It's only when stress becomes distress that you have to start worrying. The stress promoted by angry, negative thoughts is distress. And where enough distress is found, disease is sure to follow.

Some stress, like some facts, comes from outside of us, and we can't do much about it. If you accidently drop a hammer on your toe, for example, it hurts and you're distressed. Hammer-on-toe-causing-pain is a distressing fact. But you have a choice. You can get mad, yell and scream, and increase your distress. You can turn your feelings inward, seeing the accident as another example of how unfair life is, and thereby also increase your distress. Or you can limit your distress by accepting the pain and making it a point to be more careful in the future.

Medical researchers have looked at the way people tend to view potentially distressful events and have designated three general categories: Type A, B and C personalities. I like to call these groups Stress Seekers (Type A), Stress Phobics (Type C) and Stress Handlers (Type B).

Stress Seekers

Stress seekers are hard-driving, volatile, success-oriented people. Eyes glued to their watch, they rush from appointment to appointment, task to task, eager to take on more responsibility. Not valuing their accomplishments for themselves, stress seekers constantly try to outdo themselves in order to make others respect and admire them. Stress seekers feel uncomfortable unless they're working hard to get ahead. And they usually have no hobbies—that's a waste of time.

What they do have, however, is a quick temper and a great deal of free-floating hostility. Stress seekers interpret most facts as a challenge. Revving up their body chemistry at inappropriate times, they're prepared to fight over every little issue.

Stress seekers are supremely competitive: they have to win, even if they're only competing against themselves. They talk fast, walk fast, drive fast, work fast and eat fast, pushing themselves to their limit and beyond.

Always on edge, angry with themselves or others, stress seekers fill their minds with angry, urgent, impatient thoughts.

Stress Seekers are Looking for Trouble

If you're a stress seeker, it doesn't take much to trigger your stress response. An angry thought, a glance at a clock, a look at the freeway traffic and the chemical fireworks begin. Highly charged chemicals get your heart beating faster and more vigorously, raise your blood pressure and increase the number of circulating blood cells. Muscle tension and strength increase; pupils dilate for better vision. Blood sugar rises, making more energy available.

These changes occur almost instantaneously as the stress seeker prepares to fight off threats to his or her life. But how do you fight off traffic? You can't punch your boss when you're told that your work is unsatisfactory. You can't smash your watch because you're late for an appointment. Are you going to take an ax to the car that backfired and woke you up? So the high-voltage chemicals flooding your body are useless worse than useless, in fact. With no outlet for their energy, they turn on you, jolting various parts of your "doctor within." If that keeps up, you will eventually blow a fuse.

Are You a Stress Seeker?

Many people are unknowingly stress seekers. Take this quick quiz to see if you have stress-seeking tendencies.

Check off the items that apply. Do you ...

( ) Speak rapidly, rushing your speech?
( ) Interrupt other people when they speak?
( ) Wolf down your meals?
( ) Detest "wasting time"?
( ) Become impatient if others are too slow?
( ) Never seem to catch up?
( ) Schedule more things than you have time for?
( ) Drive too fast, even if you're not late?
( ) Shun intimate relationships because they take time from your career, or because they seem like a waste of time and energy?
( ) Always want to win, even when playing with your child?
( ) Leave very little time for rest, relaxation and enjoyment?

The more items you checked, the more likely it is that you're a stress seeker. Even checking only one item can suggest trouble. Your mind is probably filled with "hurry" and "more" and "better" and "harder" and "out of my way" and "can't you speed up?," and "why are you holding me back?" Your biochemical assembly lines are working overtime to manufacture enough of the high-voltage chemicals required to keep your mind and body racing at full speed. And your heart, thymus, adrenal glands and other parts of your body may be already suffering the consequences.

A Lesson from the Laboratory

An interesting study demonstrated what happens when the powerful stress hormones are released too often. A group of rats was forced to listen to a tape recording of a cats chasing rats, complete with hissing and squealing. Stress chemicals flooded the rats' bodies as they prepared to fight or run away from the cat. But the cat was imaginary, nothing more than a recording. Like the stress seeker at work, at home and in traffic, the rats were preparing for a battle they would not, and could not, fight. Eventually, the stress wore out their "doctor within;" and many of the rats died. Autopsies showed that they had suffered from death of heart tissue. There had been no cat threatening them; their reaction was based solely on their perception of the fact.

We think we're smarter than animals, but we make the same mistakes the rats did. In fact, our mistakes are worse, because we're supposed to know better. The rats couldn't know it was only a recording they were hearing; they couldn't help turning on their stress response at the wrong time. But we should know better than to respond as stress seekers when we're caught in traffic, when the boss promotes someone else or when a police officer gives us a ticket.

Remember: Your interpretation of the facts determines your thoughts. Thoughts can create or add to stress and stress will sabotage your "doctor within."

Stress Seeking: A Case History

John R. is a 35-year-old stress seeker with a good job in the aerospace industry. He lives in a beach town near Los Angeles and drives into Beverly Hills to see me once a year for a checkup. A few months ago we had an unscheduled meeting in the hospital. John had been upset when he didn't get a promotion he thought he deserved. Instead of talking it over with his supervisors, he threw a tantrum, then stomped out, hopped in his car and headed north on Pacific Coast Highway. The California Highway Patrol stopped him because he was going 80 miles an hour. John argued with the patrol officer and wound up in jail. It was while telling off his cellmate that he suffered the chest pains that sent him to the hospital.

I had explained the relationship between stress seeking and heart disease to him several times. He never paid attention. This time he took very careful notes. Since that time, John has worked very hard to control himself. "I'm in no hurry to die, Arnie," he said.

Stress Phobias

Stress phobics are the opposite of stress seekers. A phobia is an irrational fear, and stress phobics have a tremendous fear of confrontations indeed, of life itself.

Stress phobics suffer in silence rather than assert themselves. They turn their anger and frustration inward. This is manifested clinically as depression. Stress phobics see the world as an unfriendly, unhappy and frightening place. These depressed stress phobics have strong feelings of hopelessness and helplessness. Nothing seems worthwhile.

The negative thoughts in their heads are turned into hormones that actually attack and suppress their immune system, making them more susceptible to disease. Stress phobics seem to have more arthritis and cancer than do stress seekers or stress handlers.

Are You a Stress Phobic?

Are you a stress phobic? Check off the items that apply to you. Do you . . .

( ) Have difficulty expressing your feelings?
( ) Feel helpless to change your personal or work situation?
( ) Accept things even if you know you could improve them?
( ) Wish that once, just once, they would listen to you?
( ) Have vague feelings of dissatisfaction?
( ) Put up with things because you're afraid they'll get worse if you try to change them?
( ) Often wonder if suicide might not be a good way to end your problems?
( ) Figure you're never going to amount to much?
( ) Have trouble picturing yourself as a successful person?
( ) Wonder if anyone would notice if you died?
( ) Wonder why you were ever born?

If you checked more than two items, you may be a stress phobic. Your mind is stuffed with "impossible" and "I can't" and "why bother" and "no one cares." These thoughts are turned into chemicals that handcuff your "doctor within" by suppressing your immune system. Your negative thoughts actually make you more vulnerable to disease. And diseased you will be unless you learn how to keep your mind clear of immune-suppressive thoughts.

Stress Phobics Invite Cancer

If you talk to cancer patients, you'll find that 70 to 75 percent of them experienced severe feelings of hopelessness, helplessness, frustration and/or inability to cope one to two years before their cancer was diagnosed. These feelings released the powerful immune-suppressing chemicals that allow cancer to flourish.

It's well known that after the death of a spouse, the widow or widower's immune system often weakens and falls, hitting rock bottom in about six months. Another six months pass, on the average, before the immune system returns to normal. What cripples the immune system? Not the fact that a spouse has died, but inconsolable grief, the guilt and the feelings of helplessness and hopelessness we sometimes feel in the wake of a death.

A Typical Stress Phobic

Steve is a typical stress phobic. He came to see me suffering from ulcerative colitis, with rectal bleeding and general abdominal discomfort. This young man, who ran a retail clothing outlet for a major manufacturer, was frustrated by company regulations. "The damn rules get in the way. I could sell more if they let me run the place my way," he complained.

When I asked him if he had explained this to upper management, he mumbled something about their not understanding. Then he admitted he was too inhibited to "make waves." Instead, he turned his anger and frustration inward, becoming depressed. He felt useless, nothing more than a cog in the company machinery.

He had no goals, nothing to look forward to. He told me that what he really wanted was to work in the company's publicity department. He took no steps to achieve that goal, however, because he felt he wasn't good enough to make it. That only increased his frustration and sense of worthlessness. Those unhappy thoughts were converted into chemical messages inside his head. These unhappy messages weakened his "doctor within" resulting in the ulcerative colitis.

An 18-year-old named Fred was another stress phobic I treated. He was in the hospital with marked anemia and weakness due to severe intestinal bleeding, diarrhea, abdominal pain and gas.

I met Fred's father in the hospital one day. A very strong-willed man who ran a rubbish collecting company, he wanted Fred to take over the business. Fred wanted to be a poet, but couldn't tell that to his father. Every time Fred went to work at the rubbish company, he developed increasing symptoms of bleeding. Feeling weak and lost, he unknowingly turned the feelings he couldn't express into a painful and dangerous illness.

Feelings that had no outlet turned on Steve and Fred, making them sick. Again, it was their interpretation of the facts that mattered. A stress seeker in their shoes would have geared up his body for a fight, not retreated inward. In either case, of course, the result is trouble.

Stress Handlers

It's the third group, called stress handlers, who seem instinctively to know how to deal with stress. As a moderator at the Second International Symposium on the Management on Stress, in 1979, I introduced a man who summed up the stress handler's approach, saying, "Don't sweat the little things. And just about everything in life is little. If you can't flee and you can't fight, then flow with it."

Stress handlers realize that most things in life aren't worth getting upset about. If the occasion demands, however, they can stand up for themselves. And if they can't resolve a problem, they learn to live with it by changing their perception of the facts.

Let's say the neighbor runs her noisy electric lawn mower every Saturday at 6 A.M. The stress seeker will jump out of bed, stomp out of the house and heart pounding, muscles tense and blood pressure sky-high angrily confront the rude neighbor. If the woman refuses to turn the machine off, the stress seeker will threaten to call the police, call his lawyer, run his own lawn mower at 5 A.M., and so on. For the stress seeker, the situation is a battle that must be won at all costs. His blood pressure will top the charts, and stress hormones will flood his body until he winsor his "doctor within" gives out.

A stress phobic will react to the same situation by turning his anger inward, bemoaning his inability to resolve the situation. Every time he hears the lawn mower he'll be reminded of his helplessness. These thoughts will slowly wear away at his immune system, making him more susceptible to disease.

Stress handlers, however, will calmly discuss the problem with the neighbor, tell a few jokes, and maybe work out a compromise. They'll make every effort to resolve the situation and keep the peace. The stress handler may be forced to handle the situation through the legal system. But, if it turns out there's no way to make the neighbor stop, the stress handler will change his perception of the facts by deciding it's a good idea to get up early and go jogging or read the newspaper while the lawn mower is running next door. In other words, the stress handler will not allow himself or herself to become sick over a lawn mower, or any other problem.

Stress handlers subconsciously know that the most important thing in life is their good health and happiness. They want to keep their endorphins and other good biochemicals flowing in goodly amounts. And they do. Stress handlers tend to be healthier than stress seekers or stress phobics because they keep their body chemistry in balance. Stress seekers may push and push until they win the point, but stress handlers are the ultimate winners: they keep their health and happiness.

Are You a Stress Handler?

Are you a stress handler? Check off the items that apply to you. Do you ...

( ) Give yourself extra time to get places, so you don't have to rush around?

( ) Go through the day at a comfortable pace, without feeling like you're always behind schedule?

( ) Sometimes enjoy a scenic detour from your usual route to work, school or home, even if it takes a little longer?

( ) Often do things, like singing or skipping, just for the fun of it?

( ) Take other's errors and omissions in stride, correcting them when necessary, but not becoming unduly upset?

( ) Take time for traditions, fantasies and rituals, and celebrate birthdays and holidays?

( ) Enjoy relationships just for their own sake?

( ) Feel you can express your feelings reasonably well with your friends, family and colleagues at work?

( ) Feel you can stand up for yourself if necessary?

( ) Firmly yet gently try to change things that you would like see changed?

( ) Find yourself accepting of those things you cannot change?

( ) Have you set reasonable goals for yourself?

( ) See yourself as a success or as someone who is working toward success?

( ) Feel reasonably satisfied with yourself?

Checking almost all or all of the above items means you are probably a stress handler. That means you're not jolting your "doctor within" with the high voltage chemicals the stress seeker inflicts on himself. Neither are you suppressing your immune system by filling your mind with stress-phobic thoughts.

A Tip from Stress Handlers

We're not all stress handlers, but we can borrow some of their techniques. The key is learning to moderate our thoughts. Stress seekers can learn to choose their battles carefully. Stress phobics, on the other hand, can become more assertive and learn to express their feelings. Moderation is the goal. Perhaps you can't become a complete stress handler, but adapting even a few stress-handling techniques can boost your "doctor within."

We'd all like to be stress handlers: relaxed, calm, able to rise to the occasion when necessary, learning to live with what we cannot change. Unfortunately, true stress handlers are a rare breed. So I propose an additional type of personality called the reformed stress seeker, a person who has learned to moderate his or her view of life.

Reformed Stress Seekers

Some years ago I was invited to speak on a radio show with Lendon Smith, M.D., the famous pediatrician. Lendon spoke about caring for infants, while I talked about stress seekers, avoiders and handlers. Naturally, one of the callers we spoke with asked how a stress seeker can become a stress handler. That's very difficult, I explained, because a stress seeker is like a race horse, straining against the reins to win every race. When they try to behave like stress handlers, they feel as if they're chained to the starting gate, unable to run. Through my own experience, and that of many of my patients, I've found that many stress seekers cannot become stress handlers anymore than a race horse can be transformed into a turtle. But they can become reformed stress seekers.

The reformed stress seeker combines the stress seeker's abundant energy and desire with the stress handler's relaxed, friendly approach. I am a reformed stress seeker. I had to learn to recognize my own stress-seeking habits, how I was feeding on them and how they hurt me. Like any compulsive person, I must always work against my stress-seeking tendencies.

Reformed stress seekers love challenges but have learned what their limits are. They'll tackle problems head-on, but if they can't lick them without making themselves sick, they'll either learn to live with it by changing their perceptions or walk away from the situation.

Lacking the stress handler's instinctive recognition of stressful situations, the reformed stress seeker must pay careful attention to his or her life, carefully assessing feelings and the environment, "sniffing out" potential stress.

Most importantly, the reformed stress seeker must decide that health and happiness are too precious to risk on unnecessary battles.

Stress Seeker Dos and Don'ts

Stress seekers must learn to slow down and calm down, to put things into perspective. Here are some guidelines:

1. Slow down the pace of your life; even a little bit will help. Learn to walk more leisurely, talk a bit slower, chew your food longer, and drive in the slow lane.
2. Set aside time *every day* for relaxation, meditation and exercise. The little time you invest in this way will pay you handsome dividends in years to come.
3. Don't try to do more than one thing at a time. Nothing is that important.
4. Don't plan to do more in a day than you can comfortably accomplish. If you finish early, go home and relax. Don't take on new responsibilities that will overload your schedule.
5. On your way to work, to the market, or anywhere, take some time to appreciate the beauty of the scenery: the sky, the people, the architecture.

6. Spend time with your loved ones and friends. Holidays, birthdays, anniversaries and graduations are great opportunities for fun.
7. Leave ten minutes early, no matter where you're going. Now you won't have to drive with an eye on the clock, fretting about being late.
8. If you find yourself too busy to do everything, you're trying to do too much. Get someone else to do it or leave it undone until tomorrow, or the next day.
9. Don't always volunteer to take on more work, go to more classes or supervise more people. If you have the time and energy, fine. If not, skip it.
10. If your work environment is constantly pressuring you, it may be time for you to look for a new job.
11. If you can't seem to finish everything you want to, learn to live with it. Remember: the only thing that is completely finished is a corpse.

Stress Phobic Dos and Don'ts

Stress phobics must learn to like and respect themselves and to appreciate their talents and potentials. Here are a few guidelines for the stress phobic:

1. Begin by admitting to yourself that you have feelings, that you're not without emotions.
2. At the start of each day, face yourself in the mirror. Acknowledge your problems and your feelings. Tell yourself what positive steps you're going to take to handle a problem and how good you feel now that you've made the decision to change.
3. Look at yourself in the mirror and tell yourself how enthusiastic you feel that you walk, talk and behave enthusiastically. Keep that spirited feeling with you all day. It will help you generate endorphins and other good biochemicals, and overcome obstacles.
4. Believe and act as if you are someone with worthwhile opinions and attitudes. You are. You are someone who deserves to be heard. Seek and you'll find the method that will enable you to be heard.

5. Learn to speak up when you feel put upon. Gently but firmly pursue your goal. Your friends will have more respect for you when you assert yourself. Gather up the facts necessary to present your side of a discussion and state them in plain language. You'll feel better when you express yourself; it's a healing feeling.
6. Look for the opportunities that are present in your life to make beneficial changes. You aren't fated to have poor health or to live in poverty. You are destined for optimal health and prosperity, and you must tell yourself so, believe it's so and act upon that belief.
7. Learn to ferret out the causes of dissatisfaction in your life. Face them. Take the steps necessary to correct them, or learn to accept what you cannot change. In any case, get going with your life.
8. Learn to like yourself. The steps that follow will help you develop a sense of self-respect and worth.
9. If you're not sure of your purpose in life, don't worry. It will come to you eventually. In the meantime, get on with your life; for life is to be lived.

Melding Mind and Body

The stress-seeking or stress-phobic mind that's filled with angry and unhappy thoughts is at odds with the rest of the body. The body desires health, but the mind keeps sending out disease-causing chemicals that attack the "doctor within" and destroy health.

The cure begins by taking the steps I've described to rid your mind of the negative thoughts that have been making you sick. Having done that, it's time to meld the mind and body into a single entity under the direction of your "doctor within," dedicated to making you healthy and happy.

How do you meld mind and body? Begin with affirmations.

Saying It Makes It So

Affirmations are strong, positive thoughts that you deliberately place in your mind. An affirmation is a way of directing your subconscious to help you achieve your goals. Positive, affirmative thoughts eliminate the negative notions that turn your mind against your body.

Affirmations are short statements you say in your head or out loud, affirming that your life is worthwhile and that you a success. With affirmations the future is already here: you tell yourself that you already have what you want.

1. Affirmations are verbal pictures of the events you want to occur.
2. Affirmations are spoken instructions to your subconscious mind.
3. Affirmations declare that you believe in yourself.
4. Affirmations affirm that what you want to happen is already happening.
5. Affirmations assert only the positive.
6. Affirmations steer your thoughts in the right direction.
7. Affirmations are a method of predisposing yourself to health and success.

Do affirmations work? That all depends on you.

Thoughts pass through our mind constantly. Most of the time we're not even aware of them. What kind of person we are depends on what sort of thoughts we hold in our minds. If we entertain greedy and evil thoughts, we will undoubtedly become greedy and evil. If we think of ourselves as sickly, we will become ill. If we meditate upon hate and revenge, we will spend our lives hateful and unhappy. But if our minds are blessed with happy, positive thoughts, we are well along the road to health and happiness.

Affirmations are strong tools for shaping your beliefs and thoughts, for making you into the person you want to be. They are a powerful medicine for mind and body.

Here are some examples of the affirmations I give my patients. As you can see, they need not be poetic or "deep." A plain and simple, positively-charged statement is all it takes. Use these affirmations, and feel free to change them to fit your needs.

Affirmation for Happiness

Many of the patients I see, regardless of their symptoms, are unhappy. I give them this happiness affirmation:

> I really like myself. I am a worthwhile person. I am joyfully happy.

Affirmation for Forgiveness

Unhappiness is often associated with grudges and hatreds. Some of the unhappiest people I've ever met have excellent memories. They can tell you every little wrong that someone ever did to them. They remember all the hurts and wounds of life and what somebody said about them 20 or 30 years ago. Some are still mad at people who are long dead. I tell them to forgive and forget. It doesn't matter what happened to you. Forgive the person, and get those hateful thoughts out of your head. By the way, you don't have to tell the person you forgive them, and you don't have to love them. Just let go of the negative thoughts. Here's what to say:

> Beginning right now, I freely and willingly forgive everyone who has ever harmed or slighted me. I happily throw away any grudges and hatreds I may carry. I also forgive myself for all the mistakes I have made. Each day I start anew, at peace with the world and at peace with myself.

Affirmation for Serenity

We could all use serenity, especially the stress seekers who are always running at top speed. Say to yourself:

I am calm, serene and have peace of mind. All
my thoughts are loving and happy. My positive
thoughts give me strength and confidence,
happiness and peace. I have the energy, time,
money and wisdom I need right now to make
my world a happy place.

Affirmation for Success

Affirmations for success are especially helpful for stress
phobics and others who feel frustrated at work, school
or life in general:

I am now happily successful. I see myself
continually achieving more success, step by step,
overcoming all obstacles. I see and feel myself
to be a successful person. I give myself the power
and permission to be a success.

Affirmation for Self-Respect

Along with success affirmations, this affirmation for self-
respect is important for stress phobics, who have so much
self-doubt and so little love for themselves:

I truly like myself. I am an interesting, energetic
man/woman who is respected and admired. I
radiate positive, friendly feelings to everyone I
meet or talk to.

The point is not to become an egomaniac but to
recognize the good qualities you have. You can be proud
of yourself without being egotistical.

Affirmation for Stress Phobics

The stress phobic must snap out of his or her depression
before progress can be made in dealing with fears of
confrontation, rejection and failure. All the affirmations,
especially those for happiness, success and self-respect,

should be repeated over and over again every day. This affirmation, too, should be a part of the stress phobic's daily regimen:

> All things are now working together for health, happiness, success and love in my life. Each morning is the start of an exciting new day, a fresh new look at the world. Every day brings more opportunities for me to assert myself and make my world a wonderful place to be.

To help build confidence in their ability to deal with the stresses of everyday life, I often give this affirmation to my stress-phobic patients:

> I am a confident and extremely capable person. People really respect and like me. I have interesting, worthwhile and challenging goals. I am a success!

Seeing It with Visualizations

Hand in hand with affirmations goes visualization. While affirmations are spoken instructions you give your mind, visualizations are mental pictures that allow you to see yourself as you want to be.

Set aside 10 to 20 minutes a day. Find a room or place where you will not be disturbed. Make yourself comfortable. Close your eyes. Let your mind's eye see yourself acting, feeling, doing, having and being what you want yourself to do, feel, have and be. Picture yourself remaining calm in a tense situation. Imagine that you're walking away from an argument. If you're a stress phobic, visualize yourself standing up calmly for your rights. Those of you on a diet can see and feel yourself 20 pounds lighter, happily and easily refusing a proffered piece of cake.

Put the words and pictures together by combining visualizations and affirmations. Say it, see it and feel it in your mind and body. Say, see and feel yourself having and being what you deserve to have and be.

With visualizations and affirmations, any positive

situation you desire can be etched into your subconscious mind and made a part of your behavior.

Seeing, Saying and Feeling It

"You know, Dr. Fox" a patient said to me, "this visualization and affirmation stuff sounds suspiciously like positive thinking."

Yes and no. Positive thinking is saying it, either out loud or in your mind. I combine that with seeing it and feeling yourself already being, doing and having all the good things you desire. The combination of affirmations, visualization and positive thinking mobilizes the endorphins and other biochemicals to help give you the good feelings, enthusiasm, energy and health you need to be a success. Perhaps the greatest medical discovery ever made is the realization that we can change our lives by changing our thoughts. We don't fully understand this process not yet but we know it works.

Most people fail in life because they've predisposed themselves to failure; they've stuffed their minds full of "I can't," "it won't work," "impossible," "it's too hard," "I'm not good enough." All these thoughts are negative affirmations, or negations, as I call them. Negations are just as powerful as affirmations are. Negative thinking cripples the mind as surely as polio cripples the body. But there's a cure for negative thinking: positive thinking.

Doc's Special Medicine

Let me tell you the story of "Doc," a middle aged messenger who believed in positive thinking. A little man without money, advanced schooling, influence or marketable skills, he used positive thinking to save lives.

He was fascinated by positive sayings, and he wrote his inspirational mottoes on slips of paper and carried them in his pocket. Everyone who received a message from him also got a slogan: "Chin up," "Take it easy," or "Tomorrow is another day."

When World War II broke out, he tried to enlist but was turned down. So he volunteered to work in a government hospital carrying bedpans, making beds, pushing carts through the corridors. He didn't mind the hard work and long hours, but he felt helpless every time he saw a soldier die. He wanted to help, but what could he do? He had no medical skills, no magic powers. One night he had an inspiration: he would save the men with positive thinking!

The next morning everyone was surprised to see the words "NOBODY DIES IN THIS WARD" written in large, bold letters on the wall. The administration was outraged and wanted to fire Doc, but the doctors and nurses saw what was happening on the ward: the power of positive thinking was taking hold. Patients were sitting up in bed, laughing and talking about the slogan, calling it medicine's "secret weapon." Some were even making bets over which of them would live the longest. A new will to live spread like wildfire through the ward. What most thought was a joke became deadly serious in the months that followed. Each patient in the ward was made to understand that he couldn't die—Doc wouldn't let him. He told them they must fight to stay alive, or the magic spell created by the words would be broken. And they lived!

Eventually, of course, some men finally died. But not with the same frequency as before the sign went up.

An Old New Idea

Positive belief is an ancient concept. In the Scriptures we read: According to your belief is it done to you. I used to wonder about that. According to your belief in what? Now I understand it to mean according to your belief in *yourself*. Success, and failure, begin with your own beliefs.

The Roman emperor Marcus Aurelius believed that "our lives are what our thoughts make of it." More recently, Frank Lloyd Wright said: "The thing always happens that you believe in. And the belief is a thing that makes it

happen. And I think nothing will happen until you /
thoroughly and deeply believe in it.

"I tell my patients that if they fill their heads with
negations, they cannot help but be failures: failures on
the job, in personal relationships and in health. But if they
prime themselves with positive thinking, affirmations and
visualizations, they are well along the road to success.

Put a positive goal in your mind; see it in your mind's
eye. Think of yourself as having already achieved the goal.
Feel those winning feelings. Now you're ready to be
successful.

Make affirmations and visualization a daily habit. You
can use some of the affirmations in this chapter, or devise
your own. Say your affirmations 50, 100 times a day you
can't overdo it. As you say them, visualize yourself being
or doing what you want to do or be. Write your affirmations
on a card and carry it with you. Look at that card often,
and repeat your affirmations silently. You can say your
affirmations any time, any place. While driving through
the inevitable traffic on the way to the office, I say my
affirmation on serenity.

Repeat your affirmations in the morning, afternoon,
evening and night. Say them quietly, with feeling; say them
loudly, with enthusiasm. I like to repeat my affirmations
over and over in my head when I'm exercising. It doesn't
matter when or where you do them, as long as you mean
them!

What's Your Outlook on Life?

Do you see the world as a happy place? Or do you view
life as a grind, unpleasant and even downright miserable?
Take the Outlook-on-Life quiz in the Immune for Life
Workbook in Chapter 7. This quiz will start you thinking
about your feelings toward yourself, others and your place
in life. The results can be used to help you determine
which of the Nutri-Prevention supplement programs may
be best suited to your needs.

"You've Got to Turn It Off!"

A 33-year-old man came to see me because he was depressed, irritable and had many aches and pains. He slept poorly and had little interest in his work, his wife or his hobbies. "Business is terrible" he told me. "I sit by the phone all day and twiddle my thumbs, waiting for it to ring."

The physical examination and laboratory tests revealed no medical problems. It was clear, however, that he had a very negative attitude toward himself, his business, his wife, and life in general. Since his lack of business seemed to bother him the most, I gave him a success affirmation.

"When you wake up in the morning" I told him, "I want you to say: 'I've got so much work I can't handle it! I love my work!' And I want you to see and feel yourself as having all that work".

He looked at me like I was crazy. "Listen, Arnold" he said, "I sit on my hands all day. My tools are getting rusty. I do all my jobs in two hours, then I sit around waiting for the phone to ring."

"Nevertheless" I answered, "I want you to say it 50, 60 times a day: 'I've got so much business I can't handle it all!' Say it, see it and feel it."

He agreed to write the affirmation down on a card, tape the card to his phone and repeat the affirmation 50 times a day. But he didn't seem to have much faith in the idea. When he left, I wondered if I would ever see him again.

A few months later he came back to my office and said, with a big grin, "Doc, you've got to turn it off! I've got so much business I can't handle it. This affirmation stuff really works! Look, when I left here last time I was going to find a real doctor who would give me some real medicine. But I said the affirmation anyway, and I'll be damned if it didn't change my attitude. I started saying and visualizing that I had lots of customers and was happy. I guess my good attitude rubbed off on my customers, because they called me more and more and told their friends about me. The more business I got, the better I felt, and the more I affirmed, the more business I got!''

A Curse No More

Another affirmation success story involved a beautiful woman who came to my office complaining of fatigue, dizziness, weakness and nausea. There was no physical cause for her problems, but it was obvious that she was very unhappy.

When I asked her about her personal life, she held her face in her hands and told me she had been through two disastrous marriages and various unhappy love affairs. "No one ever looks past my face and body" she said. "My beauty is a curse."

Explaining that I felt her symptoms were caused by negative thoughts, I asked her to say this affirmation several times a day: "This is the beginning of a wonderful new day for me. What I do today is important. When tomorrow comes this day will be gone, leaving behind whatever I have traded for it. I pledge to myself that this day shall be for good, for gain, for happiness and success."

"Okay," she said, listlessly. "I'll try it."

Three weeks later she bounced jubilantly into my office and said, "It worked! I said it every day, ten times a day. I got everyone in my office to say it with me, too. We stand in a circle every morning and hold hands when we say it. We're all feeling better. It's like we all share a secret medicine. It's changed my whole attitude. I want every day to be a good day. I won't let anything stand in the way of my good day."

I see this woman once a year now, for her regular checkup. Her personal life is running smoothly now. She's in good shape, not only physically but emotionally and spiritually as well.

Now It's Up to You

When the examination is complete and all the impressions

and data have been collected and evaluated, I sit down with a patient to begin summing up. The patient is given copies of my findings and impressions, test results and other information. We review the material, and I explain the various options or programs I have worked out to enhance their health. We meet again to review their progress and fine-tune their health program, if necessary.

My friends, you're at the same point as my patients: you're at a crucial turning point in your life. You've learned about your "doctor within," the immune system, Super Foods, affirmations, stress handling, "wogging" and more. You've digested the ins and outs of the Immune for Life program. I've given you the information: the rest is up to you.

I could write a library of books on the immune system and the "doctor within." But all the words, arguments, principles, lists and diagrams in the world won't do a bit of good until you decide to take the steps necessary to protect and strengthen your "doctor within." I've given you the pieces; it's up to you to assemble them into a beautiful picture of lifelong health and happiness.

Yes, you may have to make many changes in your diet, your outlook on life, your exercise habits and so on, and that can be intimidating. I tell my patients to take it one day at a time. For example, every time you sit down to eat, think about how food helps or hurts you. Are there Super Foods on your plate? Which items should be removed from your diet? Which healthy foods can you eat instead? When you feel yourself becoming angry, ask yourself if this blowup is absolutely necessary for your safety and well-being. Review your progress before going to bed at night. Have you improved your diet? Are you becoming more of a stress handler? Did you exercise vigorously today? If you've made strides today, pat yourself on the back. If not, don't get upset. Remind yourself that the changes I'm advising you to make are vital, and think of ways to make tomorrow a positive day for your health and happiness.

Years ago I spent a great deal of time explaining the "doctor within," Super Foods, and so on, to a patient of mine, a well-known sports figure. He was suffering from frequent colds and a depressed immune system. He listened very carefully, asked intelligent questions and took careful notes. He came back to see me periodically, each time assuring me that he was following the program I had outlined for him. But I could tell from the examinations that his health was disintegrating. His laboratory tests and other clues told me that he wasn't following my advice. His wife called me one day to say that he hadn't made any changes in his diet or his outlook. Indeed, she said, he continued to eat all the wrong foods and did nothing to alleviate his stress. This man practiced a form of denial, and he eventually wound up with cancer.

Let me tell you about another patient, a man with diabetes, which required daily insulin injections. This wealthy businessman loved to eat large, thick steaks, sweet-and-sour Chinese food and deli-sandwiches. He ate his way through the fanciest restaurants in Los Angeles and, for that matter, all over the U.S., as he traveled about the country. He came to see me regularly, listening attentively as I explained how and why he should start protecting his "doctor within." Like the sports figure, however, he didn't make the commitment to his health. Then a diabetes-related gangrene attacked his foot, and part of it had to be amputated. Now he was ready to make the changes. Unlike a salamander, he couldn't grow back the part of his foot he had lost. But by adopting all the health-enhancement techniques I've described in this book, and others that I designed specifically for him, he brought his diabetes under control. He is doing well, feels well and is looking forward to many productive and healthy years.

I can't slap your hand every time you reach for unhealthy food; I can't force you to follow the Immune for Life program. But I can tell you that there is no more precious thing on earth than your good health. Nature has endowed you with the best doctor you can have: your "doctor within." As a physician, my advice is to take care of it. You'll be rewarded with long life, vibrant health and happiness.

Rx for Enthusiasm!

Before you read through the rest of the book and embark on the Immune for Life program, I'd like to leave you with a final thought that may help you, not only with the program but with every other part of your life as well. That, my friend, is enthusiasm. Whatever you do, do it with enthusiasm. There's nothing like joyous exuberance to raise your endorphins and brighten your outlook. We can all use a generous dose of sparkling joie de vivre.

Here's a prescription I give my patients: a prescription for enthusiasm. I encourage all of my patients, even those who are happy and healthy, to add this to their lives.

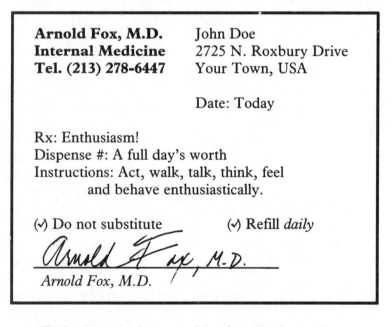

Arnold Fox, M.D.	John Doe
Internal Medicine	2725 N. Roxbury Drive
Tel. (213) 278-6447	Your Town, USA

Date: Today

Rx: Enthusiasm!
Dispense #: A full day's worth
Instructions: Act, walk, talk, think, feel
    and behave enthusiastically.

(✓) Do not substitute   (✓) Refill *daily*

Arnold F ox, M.D.

Enthusiasm is the extra bit of magic that makes your affirmations and visualizations even more powerful. It's well known that thinking enthusiastically can make the most depressed person feel elated, excited and optimistic. I tell my patients to look into the mirror every morning and tell themselves that they are enthusiastic! That they walk, talk and act enthusiastically, and that they feel enthusiastic.

It's a great prescription, and it really works. For best results, use it over and over again. Enthusiasm is nontoxic and has no harmful side effects.

If you fill this prescription in the pharmacy of your mind, and fill it correctly, you will begin to feel better. Physical problems may require other prescriptions, but we can always benefit from extra enthusiasm. You'll be rewarded with endorphins and the other good biochemicals that make you feel happy and healthy.

Through the years, having treated thousands of patients suffering from a wide variety of diseases, I have seen what a powerful medicine the positive, determined mind can be. I can tell you that happy thoughts are a tremendous shot in the arm for your "doctor within." Using the "Dos and Don'ts" and affirmations in this chapter, using them with vigor and enthusiasm, will go a long way toward making you the healthy, happy and successful person you deserve to be.

Chapter 6

Special Notes

Many of my patients ask me lots of questions. I encourage them to do so, for I believe that patients should be active, informed participants in their health. Don't be afraid to ask your doctor questions. Where your health is concerned, no question is silly or trivial: every question is very important.

Let's look at some of the questions that are raised over and over in discussions with my patients.

What Is Cholesterol, and How Does It Harm Us?

Cholesterol is a fat-soluble steroid alcohol, a natural substance made in our body. We use cholesterol to help absorb and transport fatty acids, to assist in the manufacture of cortisone, sex hormones, and vitamin D, and otherwise keep the body running smoothly. Cholesterol is necessary in small amounts. The problems begin when there is too much cholesterol in your body.

Cholesterol is a major contributor to heart disease, the number one killer in this country. There are many kinds of heart disease, but coronary artery disease (CAD) is far and away the most prevalent—and excess cholesterol is a major contributor to CAD.

With CAD, the coronary arteries that supply fresh, oxygen-rich blood to the heart muscle are blocked, dammed up by cholesterol/fat plugs. Blood can no longer flow freely, and a part of the heart muscle dies from lack of blood. This is known as a heart attack. Whether the attack is mild or deadly depends on the nature and location of the coronary artery blockage. Some cases are so mild, the victim may not realize they have suffered a heart attack. Other attacks are instantly deadly. In some cases the person is forewarned by pain and/or shortness of breath. Other times, the first symptom—a massive heart attack is the last.

As deadly as CAD is, it is essentially a plumbing problem; the pipes get clogged. It may begin when a little bit of cholesterol floating through the bloodstream sticks to the wall (interior lining) of one of the coronary arteries. That's not too bad; the bit of cholesterol is small, the artery opening relatively wide. More than enough blood can get through; the flow is hardly disturbed. But the little piece of cholesterol attracts other pieces, as well as fat and cellular debris. Like a cancer, the little bit of cholesterol "grows" into a nice-size dam that slows the flow of blood through the coronary artery.

In some people, the dam keeps growing, slowly throttling the flow of blood, until heart muscle "downstream" of the blockage dies. In other cases, the blockage may not be large enough to cause an attack. But the dam slows the flow of blood, and sluggish blood is more likely to clot. If a clot forms and sticks in the dam, the result can be a sudden heart attack.

Good and Bad Cholesterol

Cholesterol is carried through the watery blood stream in different "vehicles" called HDL, LDL and VLDL. When we doctors measure out patients' cholesterol, we pay special attention to the total cholesterol (TC), the HDL, and the LDL.

TC is an important indicator of your risk of coronary artery disease. The higher your TC, the greater your risk. The average American with the average cholesterol of 220 has the average heart attack. You want to be better than average; much better. I like to see my patients keep their TC below 160. The ideal figure is 100 plus your age. (For a 42-year-old person, that would be 142.)

HDL (high density lipoprotein) is called the "good cholesterol" because it is felt to clean up the arteries, grabbing excess cholesterol off the artery walls, sending it to the liver for disposal. Thus, while keeping your TC low, you want your HDL to be high. I like to see my patients keep their HDL at 45-50 mg/dl (milligrams per deciliter) or higher. Exercise is an excellent way of raising the HDL.

Stress lowers HDL. If you smoke, here's another reason to quit: Smokers have lower levels of HDL than non-smokers (Journal of the American Medical Association, May 20, 1988).

LDL (low density lipoprotein), the "bad cholesterol," seems to be a delivery truck of sorts, helping to bring cholesterol to the artery walls where it can stick. Keep your LDL as low as possible. I like my patients to keep their LDL below 100 mg/dl.

There's another cholesterol called VLDL (very low density lipoprotein). VLDL is also considered a "bad" cholesterol. Averages for VLDL range up to 40. I like to see my patients keep their VLDL at about 20 or less.

Measuring the Risk

There are two simple indexes to help you measure your risk of coronary artery disease. They're called CADRIF 1 and CADRIF 2. CADRIF stands for Coronary Artery Disease Risk Factor. Both indexes use the total cholesterol, HDL and LDL numbers we've already discussed.

To find your CADRIF 1, divide your total cholesterol (TC) by your HDL. If your TC is 250 and your HDL is 25, your CADRIF is:

$$\frac{250}{25} = 10$$

A CADRIF 1 of 10 puts you at great risk for coronary artery disease. For the best of health, your CADRIF 1 should be less than 4.

CADRIF 2 compares your "good" and "bad" cholesterol. Again, you want the figure to be nice and low. To find your CADRIF 2, divide your LDL by your HDL. If your LDL is 190 and your HDL is 25, your CADRIF 2 is:

$$\frac{190}{25} = 8.6$$

This score also puts you at great risk of coronary artery disease. I like to see my patients keep their CADRIF 2 below 3.

What Are Your Odds?

Call your doctor, get your total cholesterol, your HDL and LDL, and figure out your CADRIFs.

CADRIF 1 = $\dfrac{\text{total cholesterol}}{\text{HDL}}$ = _____ =

CADRIF 2 = $\dfrac{\text{LDL}}{\text{HDL}}$ = _____ =

The chart below shows the standard adopted by a prominent laboratory to assess a person's risk of suffering a heart attack.

	CADRIF 1		CADRIF 2	
	Men	Women	Men	Women
1/2 the average risk	3.43	3.27	1.00	1.47
Average risk	4.97	4.44	3.55	3.22
Twice the average risk	9.55	7.05	6.25	5.03
Three times the average risk	23.39	11.04	7.99	6.14

These figures give the averages. But remember, average is awful! The average person with the average cholesterol has the average heart attack. You want to be better than average—much better. An easy way to remember what you want your CADRIF to be, for both men and women is:

CADRIF 1 - less than 4
CADRIF 2 - less than 3

Where Does Cholesterol Come From?

Our bodies make all the cholesterol we require—there is no need to eat any additional cholesterol. But eat it we do, in large amounts. Cholesterol is found in foods that come from animals: meat, fish, chicken, eggs, milk, cheese, and so on. Fruits, legumes, nuts and seeds, contain absolutely no cholesterol.

Some patients are surprised when I get their laboratory report back, and tell them that they have a high cholesterol. "But I don't eat meat, and hardly any dairy products!" they exclaim.

It turns out that many of these patients were consuming large amounts of saturated fats—often unknowingly, for saturated fats are mixed in many of our processed and restaurant foods. Saturated fats elevate your cholesterol level; a good reason to keep your saturated fat intake low.

People eating the Standard American Diet consume roughly between 600 and 1,000 milligrams (mg.) of cholesterol every day. I tell my patients that they should be taking in less than 300 mg. per day. If their cholesterol count is high, they should restrict themselves to 100 mg. a day or less.

Is it important to cut back on our cholesterol? Yes. Elevated cholesterol is a major risk factor for coronary artery disease. And the coronary arteries are not the only "pieces of plumbing" that cholesterol can clog. For example, blockages in brain arteries can cause a stroke; in the ear, deafness. Practically every patient I've seen has had a high blood cholesterol level when they first came to see me.

Dr. Fox's "Natural Stuff" to Lower Cholesterol

In my office, on radio call-in shows, at my speeches, in letters to me, even on street corners, people constantly ask me if there is something they can take to lower their cholesterol.

There are drugs to lower cholesterol, but most are not that effective and, like all drugs, they have serious side effects. Newer drugs are more effective, but still have side effects. These drugs should be reserved for the rare cases that do not respond to diet and my Natural Stuff to lower cholesterol.

I have found certain foods, supplements and fibers lower cholesterol as well as or better than the drugs, without any side effects except better overall health. Studies in the medical literature support my findings.

Of course, I tell everyone who asks that the best way to handle elevated cholesterol is to begin by switching to the Super Food Diet. The Super Food Diet is low in cholesterol and fat, but high in the complex carbohydrates which help lower cholesterol.

Here is a list of the natural substances I have used to help my patients with problem cholesterol. I don't have people take them all at once; I pick 2 or 3 that best suit their needs, lifestyles, dietary tastes, and so on. (I tell my patients to use the natural forms of these substances whenever possible.)

Oat bran: My favorite anti-cholesterol fiber. As you recall from the "Super Foods" chapter, oat bran can beat drugs when it comes to lowering cholesterol—and it has none of the drug's side effects. Like the other fibers, oat bran also provides protection against other diseases and problems.

Here's a recipe for delicious oat bran muffins.

Ingredients:

2 1/4 cups	oat bran
1 tsp.	baking powder
a handful	raisins or blueberries
	cinnamon to taste
1/2 cup	skim milk
3/4 cup	apple juice concentrate
2	egg whites

Preheat oven to 450 degrees. Mix all the ingredients together in a bowl. Add the cinnamon last, to taste. Pour mixture into a cup cake baking tin. Bake for 16 minutes.

I tell my patients with elevated cholesterol to have a bowl of oat bran for breakfast and 2 to 3 oat bran muffins during the day.

Guar gum: I usually start people on 500 milligram capsules, two to three before meals. When taken before meals, guar gum also helps reduce the appetite by filling up the belly.

Pectin capsules: also apples and other fruits containing natural pectin. I keep a bowl full of apples in the waiting room at my office, and encourage my patients to eat 2 or 3 apples a day—for pectin and many other nutrients. Pectin lowers total cholesterol and LDL (the "bad" cholesterol), and helps raise the "good" HDL. For my patients who take pectin capsules, I generally recommend two 15-grain capsules, three times a day, with meals.

Niacin (vitamin B3):   I start my patients on 250 milligram timed-release capsules, two a day, gradually increasing to 1,000 milligrams, twice a day. I warn my patients about the flushing and tingling sensations that can occur when taking niacin, and check their liver tests periodically. Taking one aspirin with the niacin generally blocks the flushing.

I personally prefer the timed disintegration capsules, but some prefer to use tablets. I have my patients who do prefer tablets begin with 50 milligrams, twice a day, gradually working up to the doses I recommend. (Most of the research was done on the tablets, but my work utilized the capsules.

Insoluble food fibers: These are natural fibers (complex carbohydrates) found in various foods, such as wheat. We do not digest and absorb these fibers. Instead, they pass through the digestive system, making the stool bulkier, more watery, and helping to speed the stool's transit through the intestines. Besides helping to lower cholesterol, food fibers help protect against cancer, as well as hemorrhoids, appendicitis, varicose veins, and other problems. Soluble fibers, such as oat bran, are better at lowering cholesterol than the insoluble fibers.

Vitamin C: Not only will vitamin C help reduce cholesterol, it has many other beneficial effects on the body.

EPA and DH: These are omega-3 fish oils that I'll talk about in the next section. I tell my patients that it is preferable to get omega-3s by eating fish, as opposed to taking fish oil supplements. If you do take fish oil supplements, keep it to the minimum.

Psyllium seeds: used in Metamucil and similar products. Studies have shown Metamucil, for example, to effectively lower total cholesterol and LDL.

Vegetables: I tell my patients with higher cholesterol that eating 5 portions of various vegetables a day will help

Meds

Noon

2:30

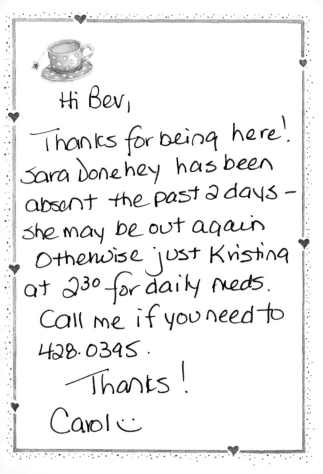

Hi Bev,

Thanks for being here!
Sara Donehey has been
absent the past 2 days -
she may be out again
  Otherwise just Kristina
at 2³⁰ for daily meds.
  Call me if you need to
428.0395.
  Thanks!
Carol ☺

lower their cholesterol. Vegetables have fiber, which helps reduce cholesterol. Researchers have isolated the active, anti-cholesterol ingredient in fiber-rich foods such as carrots, broccoli, cabbage, and onion. Calcium pectate, a part of plant cells found in these fibers, attaches itself to bile acids in the intestine and eliminates them. Since the body needs bile acids to digest fats, and since bile acids are made from cholesterol, the body must use some of its cholesterol to manufacture the bile acids. This helps reduce cholesterol. Not only that, calcium pectate helps to control the free fatty acids that may cause colon cancer. And, the more vegetable you eat, the less room you have in your stomach for the high-cholesterol meat and dairy products that are such a large part of the Standard American Diet.

Fruit: Unless there is a reason to the contrary, such as diabetes, 3, 4 or 5 servings of various fruits daily will provide ample supplies of pectin, which will help lower cholesterol.

Activated charcoal: This is a special type of charcoal— it comes in capsules—which has been used for many years in every hospital emergency room as an antidote to many poisons. I've been using it for several years for patients with elevated cholesterol. I generally have my patients work up to half a gram, twice a day, with meals. Incidently, I've been using activated charcoal for over thirty years to reduce the symptoms of excess intestinal gas.

Niacinamide: A "version" of niacin, good; but not as good as niacin at lowering cholesterol.

Some people have a genetic disposition toward high cholesterol. No matter how strict their diet, their cholesterol remains alarmingly high. In cases like these, cholesterol-lowering drugs are indicated.

For most of us, however, careful attention to diet, exercise, and some of Dr. Fox's Natural Stuff to Lower

Cholesterol is all it takes to get our cholesterol nice and low—and keep it there.

Is Fish Oil Good for You? Isn't Oil Pure Fat, and Bad for You?

When I was a child, my mother used to tell me to eat my fish: "It'll make you healthier and smarter," she would say. I didn't believe that, but I was smart enough to know that it wasn't a good idea to argue with my mother. She had a right hook any boxer would be proud of.

In the early 1970s researchers began gathering evidence suggesting that Mom was right: fish is good for you. Danish scientists noted that Eskimos living in Greenland had very little heart disease, despite the fact that they ate large amounts of fat in the form of fish, whale, and seal meat. In one study of 1,800 Eskimos, there were only three heart attacks in over twenty years. By was of comparison, there would have been more than 30 times as many heart attacks among 1,800 Americans during the same two-plus decades.

The researchers knew that when the Eskimos moved to Denmark and adopted a Western-style diet they suffered from clogged arteries and heart attacks at an increased rate. This suggested that there was something in the Eskimo diet protecting their hearts from all the fat they ate by:

- thinning their blood. "Thinner" blood flows smoothly through the arteries. It is less likely to form unnecessary blood clots that can lodge in one of the tiny coronary arteries and trigger a heart attack;
- reducing total cholesterol;
- lowering blood fat (triglyceride) levels; and
- possibly lowering LDL (the "bad" cholesterol that deposits fat along the artery walls).

That special something protecting the Eskimos from coronary heart disease turned out to be a fat (oil) contained in the fish they ate. Specifically, it was a kind of fat know as omega-3 fatty acids.

Not All Fats Are Created Equal

Although as a general rule eating too much fat is unhealthy, not all fat is the same. The fat in a steak, for example, is different from the fat in peanuts, because different fatty acids are used to put together the fats. (Fatty acids are the "building blocks" of fat, the smaller units assembled in various ways to produce different kinds of fat.)

The Eskimos ate fat which contained good amounts of omega-3 fatty acids. Our Western diet, on the other hand, contains lots of omega-6 fatty acids.

Fatty acids are grouped according to the placement of the first double bond occurring along their carbon atom "spine." "Omega-3 means that the first double bond is associated with the third carbon atom from the "omega" end of the fatty acid. In an omega-6 fatty acid, the first double bond is associated with the sixth carbon atom. Where the first double bond between carbon atoms happens to be may seem trivial, but we've learned that small variations can make a world of difference in the microscopic world of molecules.

We who eat the Standard American Diet tend to get a lot of omega-6 fatty acids in our diet. The Eskimo experience suggests that eating more omega-3s is a good idea. It's an interesting situation: One kind of fat helps protect you from the dangers of other fats. As I pointed out previously, fish are a good source of omega-3 fatty acids. Fatty fish such as Norway sardines and salmon tend to have more of the omega-3s than "skinny" fish such as albacore tuna, striped bass and Pacific halibut.

Although fatty fish have more of the protective omega-3s than to their "skinny" counterparts, I don't like to see my patients eating lots of herring. Instead, I suggest that they have two to three fish meals a week, eating different kinds of fish, and keep their total fat intake low.

By the way, studies suggest that in addition to guarding against heart disease, the omega-3s may also protect us against stroke, some autoimmune diseases, diabetes, headaches, high blood pressure and other problems.

The book on fish oil is not closed; research continues. A newly reported study conducted at the University of California at San Francisco (Internal Medicine World Report, May 1-14, 1988, p. 52) found that feeding rabbits fish oil slowed the formation of "dams" in the animals' arteries. This study supported others suggesting that the omega-3s can help prevent heart disease.

Can Aspirin Prevent Heart Attacks?

Thirty years ago I began using small amounts of aspirin, about one half an aspirin a day, for patients with what we used to call "small strokes" (now called transient ischemic attacks, or T.I.A.s). Recently, taking small doses of aspirin has been promoted as a way to protect certain people from heart disease.

Aspirin "thins out" the blood, helping the blood flow more smoothly through the arteries, and making it less likely to clot.

About four years ago I enrolled in a long-term study with some 22,000 other medical doctors. The study was designed to test whether aspirin prevented heart attacks, and to see if beta carotene (proto vitamin A) helps protect against cancer.

The study was recently halted because the results were so good, it was deemed unethical to withhold aspirin from the doctors who might need to take aspirin, but were receiving a placebo ("sugar pill") instead.

This study confirmed what we've known for a long time: Small doses of aspirin (5 grains, or 325 milligrams) can help prevent heart attacks in patients at risk of coronary artery disease.

Aspirin is even useful after a heart attack has begun. A recent study reported in the May 1, 1988 issue of "Internal Medicine World Review," involved over 17,000 patients with symptoms of a heart attack in North America, Europe, and Australia. Those who were given one-half an aspirin tablet a day for one month showed a 21% decrease in overall mortality five weeks later, enjoying continuing protection for one to two years, minimum. The risk of stroke, subsequent heart attacks and sudden cardiac (heart) death was also reduced by about a third.

Patients given a drug called streptokinase did better than those on aspirin, and the ones given aspirin plus streptokinase did best of all.

Like all drugs, aspirin has side effects. The best idea is to use the Immune for Life program to keep your arteries clean and to remain healthy.

Please do not start taking lots of aspirin! If you feel you are at risk of heart disease, or if you have any symptoms, such as chest pain or shortness of breath, see your doctor.

What Is the Single Most Important, Easily Done Test for the Immune System?

In chapter 9 I talk about T4/T8 ratio, an important index which at one time was considered the barometer of the immune system. I've found, however, that the absolute number of T4 "helper" cells is perhaps the single most important test of immune system strength. I watch the total T4 count when monitoring the immune status of patients infected with various organisms. Many doctors also use the total T4 count when measuring the benefits of AIDS treatment.

The T4 cells are the helper cells that prod the immune system to fight when bacteria, viruses or other germs invade the body. The T4s can be greatly reduced in illnesses such as AIDS.

Here's an immune system profile I use for my patients. This particular patient, a 29 year old man, complained of feeling tired, and had an enlarged gland in his neck.

	Results	Desired range
White blood cells	3,000	4,800-10,800
(our main immune fighters)		
Red blood cells	4.76 million	4.1-6.1 million
Hemoglobin	12.7 grams	13.5-18 grams
Hematocrit	38.7%	41-52%
Lymphocytes	42%	15-45%
(T and B cells)		
Neutrophils	50%	50-80%
(Immune system soldiers)		
Monocytes	8%	0-12%
("Cell eaters")		
T4 absolute	494	385-2,090
(Total number of helper cells)		
T8 absolute	403	165-1,290
(Total number of suppressor cells)		
T4/T8 ratio	1.2	1.5 or so
(compares the number of helper to suppressor cells)		

I'll talk more about these tests in Part 3, the "Immune for Life Information File." The point is, we doctors can look at several indices of immune system function by taking a simple blood test.

This young man scored low on enough tests to make me wonder. I ordered a test to check for the presence of antibodies to HIV-I (human immune) deficiency virus, formerly know as the HTLV-III).

The test was positive. It was repeated, then confirmed with a Western Blot test. The young man had AIDS.

Within a month his total T4 count had dropped to 225 as he became clinically more ill. With proper treatment, including the Immune for Life program, his T4 rose to 600, indicating that his immune system was gaining strength. His AIDS was not cured, but he was doing better.

It's been said that the wisest people are those who ask the most questions. It's also been said that if you ask you shall receive. Ask questions unending and receive all the knowledge of health and happiness you possibly can.

Part 2

The Immune for Life Workbook

Chapter 7

Measuring Immunity

You've looked at the various aspects of the Immune for Life program. Now it's time to take a look at yourself. How immune are you? Is your diet full of the Super Foods that give your "doctor within" the vitamins, minerals and other nutrients needed to fight illness and distress? Or are you eating the Standard American Diet that causes so much disease and death? Is your mind filled with positive, happy thoughts? Or are you a stress seeker or a stress phobic? Are you a regular and vigorous exerciser, or do you lie down whenever the urge to exercise comes over you?

I'm going to ask you to do some interesting work in this chapter. You'll find three quizzes that contain the same kinds of questions I ask my patients. Taking the quizzes will teach you a lot about outlook on life, exercise and nutrition, as I see it. Your scores will be used to determine which of the four Nutri-Prevention supplement programs may be right for you. And at the end of the chapter you'll find a list of immune-system laboratory tests that you should consider having performed by your physician to measure certain indicators of the immune system.

Answer all the questions honestly. No one but you needs to see what you write.

After you've been on the Immune for Life program for about two months, take the three quizzes again. You'll be surprised at how much higher you score, and how much better you feel.

Outlook-on-Life Test

What *is* your outlook on life? Is your world an interesting, enjoyable place to be, or is every day a grind? Take this quiz, circling the number below each statement that most closely describes how you feel. Keep a running total as you go through the test in the "points" column on the right.

1. Generally speaking, I consider myself to be:

enthusiastic   bored and
about life, and   uninterested
about myself.   in life.

10   9   8   7   6   5   4   3   2   1

points: _____

2. My life is:

exciting and   the same thing
fresh everyday.   over and over.

10   9   8   7   6   5   4   3   2   1

points: _____

3. I have:

lots of things I   no goals or
want to do   reasons to exist.

10   9   8   7   6   5   4   3   2   1

points: _____

4. In striving toward my goals, I have:

made very good progress.

made no pro-gress at all.

10   9   8   7   6   5   4   3   2   1

points: _____

5. As an individual, I have:

made a contribution to the world.

done nothing at all

10   9   8   7   6   5   4   3   2   1

points:_____

6. My ability to find or define meaning and purpose in my life is:

limitless.

nonexistent.

10   9   8   7   6   5   4   3   2   1

points: _____

7. When it comes to running my life, I am:

completely free to choose my destiny.

completely bound by out-side forces and by own limitations.

10   9   8   7   6   5   4   3   2   1

points: _____

8. When thinking of my life and what I have accomplished, I:

always see a   usually wonder
reason for my   why I was ever
existence.   born.

10   9   8   7   6   5   4   3   2   1

points: _____

9. If I died right now, people would say my life was:

very   completely
worthwhile.   worthless.

10   9   8   7   6   5   4   3   2   1

points: _____

10. I think of death:

rarely.   often.

10   9   8   7   6   5   4   3   2   1

points: _____

11. I have considered suicide:

never.   often.

10   9   8   7   6   5   4   3   2   1

points: _____

12. As far as job success is concerned:

it's right around   I'll never be
the corner.   successful.

10   9   8   7   6   5   4   3   2   1

points: _____

13. My personal relationships are:

enjoyable and   always miserable
worthwhile.   failures.

10   9   8   7   6   5   4   3   2   1

points: _____

14. I consider obstacles to be:

a challenge to   the reason I
overcome.   always fail.

10   9   8   7   6   5   4   3   2   1

points: _____

15. Other people:

really like me.   can't stand me.

10   9   8   7   6   5   4   3   2   1

points: _____

16. I have:

lots of friends.   no friends.

10   9   8   7   6   5   4   3   2   1

points: _____

17. I command:

a great deal of   absolutely no
respect.   respect.

10   9   8   7   6   5   4   3   2   1

                                        points: _____

18. Knowing what I know now, I would prefer:

to live my life   never to have
exactly as I   been born.
have.

10   9   8   7   6   5   4   3   2   1

                                        points: _____

19. When faced with an unfamiliar task or job, I usually:

solve the prob-   make a big deal
lem in no time.   of things.

10   9   8   7   6   5   4   3   2   1

                                        points: _____

20. My gravestone will say:

here lies a good   here lies some-
person we will   one nobody
miss.   cares about.

10   9   8   7   6   5   4   3   2   1

                                        points: _____

When I give this or any other test to my patients,
I look at their responses as part of the total bundle of

information I have gathered. I often ask more questions to clarify or expand upon a certain issue, or adjust the quiz as individual needs require. This test is another tool for evaluating a person, along with the complete medical history, physical examination, laboratory tests and other studies.

Generally speaking, if your score is below 50, your mind is filled with negative, unhappy, self-doubting thoughts. As you recall from our discussions in Chapters One and Five, an unhappy mind is mirrored by an unhealthy body.

If your total is between 50 and 100, you have a poor outlook on life. Your unhappy thoughts are probably suppressing your immune system.

Scores above 100 indicate that you have a positive outlook on life that's giving your "doctor within" a shot in the arm.

A score of 150 or more suggests that your mind is filled with happy, positive thoughts that are helping to make your "doctor within" as strong as possible.

What should you do if your score is low? Reread "Melding Mind and Body" (Chapter Five). Say your affirmations 50, 70, 100 times a day. Practice visualizations regularly. Do so until you realize, and firmly believe that you are a worthwhile person who deserves happiness and success.

Some of my patients had low scores on this test when they first came to see me. Learning to change their attitudes and habits has helped them score higher on the real test: life.

Exercise Quiz

Thanks to the determined man on the gurney I saw pulling himself, inch by inch, through the race at UCLA, I changed my attitude toward regular exercise. How do you feel about exercise and physical activity? Here's a short quiz, with questions similar to those I ask my patients, to help determine your exercise attitudes and practices. Circle the number below each question that corresponds to the statement that most closely reflects your attitude or practice. Keep a running total of your score in the "points" column.

1. I have been checked out by my physician and given the "OK" to exercise:

Yes	6
No	0

points: _____

2. I do aerobic-type exercise (such as brisk walking, jogging, running, bicycling, swimming, rowing and cross-country skiing):

Five times a week or more	6
Four times a week	5
Three times a week	4
Two times a week	3
Once a week	2
Once every ten days or so	1
Never	0

points: _____

3. I've been following an aerobic-type exercise program (brisk walking, swimming, bicycling, aerobic dancing, etc.):

Continuously for many years	6
Off and on for many years	4
I just started	3
Haven't exercised in a while	1
Never exercised	0

points: _____

4. While exercising, my heart rate is in my Heart Rate Target Zone:
(see chart on page 117)

Always	6
Occasionally	4
Rarely	2
Never	0

points: _____

5. I enjoy wogging (see page 120) 25 minutes a day, four days a week:

Yes	4
No	0

points: _____

6. I participate in games and sports such as singles tennis, racquetball, basketball or karate for fun and exercise.

Yes	4
No	0

points: _____

7. I participate in games and sports such as doubles tennis, baseball, badminton, volleyball or bowling for fun and relaxation.

Yes	4
No	0

points: _____

8. I look for ways to add steps to my days, such as parking my car a block or two from my destination

and walking the rest of the way, walking instead of driving to nearby stores or offices, etc.

Always	6
Most of the time	4
Occasionally	2
Never	0

points: _____

9. When I have to go up or down a few floors, I:

Always use the stairs	6
Often use the stairs	4
Occasionally use the stairs	3
Rarely use the stairs	1
Never use the stairs	0

points: _____

10. If I have to go less than a mile, I:

Always walk	6
Often walk	4
Occasionally walk	3
Rarely walk	1
Never walk	0

points: _____

11. On the job I am:

Very physically active	6
Fairly physically active	4
Moderately active	3
Mostly sitting down	1
Completely sedentary	0

points: _____

12. I exercise my abdominal and back muscles:

Four or more times a week	6
A couple of times a week	4
Rarely	2
Never	0

points: _____

13. I exercise my upper-body muscles (arms, chest, shoulders) by lifting light weights, doing push-ups, pull-ups, or other upper-body activities/exercises:

Four or more times a week	6
A couple of times a week	4
Rarely	2
Never	0

points: _____

14. I stretch for at least ten minutes a day:

Four or more times a week	6
Three times a week	4
Once in a while	1
Never	0

points: _____

15. When I feel the urge to exercise, I:

Exercise	6
Sometimes exercise	4
Occasionally exercise	2
Ignore the urge	0

points: _____

Scoring Your Exercise Quiz

Again, any test I give to my patients is evaluated as part of the total information I have gathered. More questions may be required to clarify or expand upon a certain issue, or to adjust the quiz as individual needs require. Taken with the complete medical history, physical examination, laboratory tests and other studies, the quiz is a good tool for evaluating a person. Generally speaking:

50 or more points is excellent.
36 to 49 is good.
20 to 35 is fair.
0 to 19 is poor.

Most of my patients would score low on this quiz. Most Americans, I believe, don't get nearly enough of the exercise their "doctor within" needs. Improving your score on this quiz is simple. All it takes is a commitment and little time. You'll be rewarded with increased health and longevity.

Nutrition Survey

Now it's time to look at what you eat to see if you're practicing the principles of the Super Food diet. Begin by keeping track of what you eat. Starting today, before you change your diet, keep a list of all the foods you eat. I explain to my patients that this is an important part of the Immune for Life process, for it allows you to see exactly what you're eating. (Many people are very surprised when they review the completed survey!) Nobody needs to know what you write here, so be very honest with yourself. The point is to learn, not to criticize. Completing this Nutrition Survey will help you take the Nutrition Quiz that follows.

Day One:

Breakfast _____

_____

Snack _____

Lunch _____

_____

Snack _____
Dinner _____

_____

Snack _____

_____

Day Two:
Breakfast _____

_____

Snack _____
Lunch _____

_____

Snack _____
Dinner _____

_____

Snack _____

Day Three:
Breakfast _____

_____

Snack _____
Lunch _____

_____

Snack _____
Dinner _____

_____

Snack _____

Day Four:
Breakfast _____

_____

Snack _____

Lunch _____

_____

Snack _____
Dinner _____

_____

Snack _____
Day Five:
Breakfast _____

_____

Snack _____
Lunch _____

_____

Snack _____
Dinner _____

_____

Snack _____
Day Six:
Breakfast _____

_____

Snack _____
Lunch _____

_____

Snack _____
Dinner _____

_____

Snack _____
Day Seven:
Breakfast _____

_____

Snack _____
Lunch _____

_____

Snack _____

Dinner _____

_____

Snack _____

List all the Super Foods you ate during the week. (See the list on page 54 if you've forgotten which are the Super Foods.) These Super Foods must be eaten fresh, not canned or pickled or swimming in oil. Neither should they be boiled to death or buried under globs of fatty sauce.

Super Foods _____

_____

_____

_____

Now list all the healthy foods you've eaten. These include any vegetables or fruits not on the Super Food list, as well as low-fat fish and nonfat dairy products. If what you ate was stored, cooked or served in an oily, fatty or sugary sauce, or was mixed with a lot of additives, it wasn't a healthy food.

Healthy Foods _____

_____

_____

Now list the not so healthy foods you've eaten. These include all the processed and packaged foods with additives, fast foods, canned fruits and vegetables packed in sugar-water, plus coffee, red meat, white bread, pasta made from white flour, packaged cereals, candy bars, cakes and pies, ice cream, etc.

Unhealthy Foods _____

_____

_____

_____

If most of your food was unhealthy, your "doctor within" is slowly but surely being crippled. But if you ate mostly Super Foods and healthy foods, you're helping your "doctor within" build super-charged health and longevity.

Nutrition Quiz

This next quiz is a learning quiz. Every time you answer a question, you'll be learning something about nutrition as I see it. The quiz will also help you to assess your dietary-nutritional status.

Circle the number of points you receive for each question, keeping track of your score in the "points" column. Start each new section with zero points. At the end of the quiz all the section totals will be added to get a grand total. The questions apply to what you generally eat. If more than one answer per question is appropriate, circle all the possibilities and average them out. If you're not sure how to answer the question, or the question doesn't apply to you, give yourself zero points.

Before I see a new patient at my office, I have him or her fill out a detailed form with questions similar to the ones you'll be answering here. Then we sit down and go over the answers. In the give-and-take of the discussion, I learn even more about his or her eating habits. My nutritionist also speaks with the patient, discovering additional diet information.

PART 1: VEGETABLES
One serving = 1/2 cup, or one medium-size vegetable

1. How many servings of fresh vegetables do you eat a day?

None	-3
One	0
Two	+1

Three   +2
Four or more   +3

points: _____

2. Do you generally eat your vegetables fresh?
No   −3
Yes   +3

points: _____

3. How many servings of vegetables from the crucifer family do you eat every day? (cabbage, cauliflower, broccoli, brussles sprouts, kohlrabi, radishes, rutabagas, etc.)
None   −3
One   +1
Two   +2
Three   +3
Four or more   +4

points: _____

4. How many servings of beta carotene-rich foods do you eat per day? (carrots, parsley, spinach, sweet potatoes, collards, kale, or other foods from beta carotene list, page 257)
None   −3
One   +1
Two   +2
Three   +3
Four or more   +4

points: _____

5. How many times a week do you eat garlic, onions, scallions (green onions), ginger or black Chinese mushrooms?

None	–3
One to two	+1
Three to five	+2
Six or more	+3

points: _____

6. Do you generally eat your vegetables:

Fried, or in a fatty, sugar or cheese sauce	–3
Boiled	–1
Baked	+1
Raw or lightly steamed	+3

points: _____

Total points for Part 1: _____

PART 2: FRUIT
One serving = 1/2 cup or one medium-size fruit

7. How many servings of fresh, raw fruits do you eat a week?

None	–3
One to four	+1
Five to seven	+2
Eight to thirteen	+3
Fourteen or more	+4

points: _____

8. Do you eat your fruits:

From a can   –3
Fresh   +3

points: _____

9. If you eat canned fruit, it is canned in:

Heavy syrup   –3
Light syrup   –1
Baked   +1
No added sugar   +1

points: _____

10. How many servings of Super Food fruit do you eat a week (peaches, cantaloupes and papayas in season)?

None   0
One   +1
Two   +2
Three   +3

points: _____

Total points for Part 2: _____

PART 3: GRAINS

One serving = one cup of cooked grain

11. How many servings of brown rice, millet, buckwheat, barley, whole-wheat bread, rolls, pasta or other whole grains do you eat weekly?

None   –1
Oned   0
Two to three   +1
Four to seven +2

Eight to thirteen   +3
Fourteen or more   +4

points: _____

12. How many servings of oat bran (including oat-bran muffins) do you eat weekly?

None   –3
One   –1
Two to three   +1
Four to six   +3
Seven or more   +4

points: _____

13. What kind of bread do you usually eat? (Circle all that apply and average.)

White bread   –2
I don't eat bread   0
Rye or pumpernickel   +1
Whole Wheat   +3

points: _____

Total points for Part 3: _____

PART 4: FISH AND CHICKEN
One serving = 3 1/2 oz.

14. How many times a week do you eat low-fat fish (cod, flounder, fresh tuna, tuna packed in water, sand dabs, sole, sea bass, red snapper, haddock, halibut)?

None   –3
One   0
Two   +2
Three or more   +3

points: _____

15. Do you have one to two servings a week of fish high in omega-3s (see page 56):

No	0
Yes	+2

points: _____

16. How many times a week do you eat chicken or turkey? (Don't count fried chicken or turkey.)

None	0
One	+1
Two	+2
Three or more	+3

points: _____

17. Do you trim away the skin and fat before cooking chicken?

Never	-3
Sometimes	-1
I don't eat poultry	0
Always	+3

points: _____

18. How do you usually prepare or eat your fish or chicken?

Fried, or baked in oil, sauce or gravy	-3
Wok-fried with a tiny bit of oil	+1
Steamed or broiled or baked without oil, sauce or gravy	+3

points: _____

Total points for Part 4: _____

PART 5: LEGUMES

19. How many servings of legumes (peas, beans, lentils) do you have a week?

None	–3
One	0
Two to three	+1
Four to seven	+2
Eight to thirteen	+3
Fourteen or more	+4

points: _____

20. How do you eat your peas?

In a sugar, cheese or butter sauce.	–3
I don't eat peas	0
Fresh, plain	+3

points: _____

21. Do you eat your beans:

In buttery or sugary sauce or with ham or other meat	–3
I don't eat beans	0
Plain, or with garlic or spices	+3

points: _____

22. How many servings of sprouted peas, beans, or lentils do you eat a week?

None	–3
One	–1
Two	+1
Three or more	+3

points: _____

Total points for Part 5: _____

PART 6: DAIRY PRODUCTS

23. How many whole eggs do you eat a week?

Seven or more	–3
Five to six	–2
Two to four	–1
None to one	0

points: _____

24. How many servings of regular-fat cheese do you eat a week?

Seven or more	–3
Five to six	–1
Two to four	–1
None to one	0

points: _____

25. Do you generally eat cheese made from skim milk?

No	–3
Yes	+3

points: _____

26. When you eat cottage cheese, is it:

Regular fat	–3
I don't eat cottage cheese	0
Low-fat	+1
Nonfat (hoop cheese)	+3

points: _____

27. When you eat yogurt, is it:

Regular fat	–3
I don't eat yogurt	0

| Low-fat | +1 |
| Nonfat, no sugar added | +3 |

points: _____

Total points for Part 6: _____

PART 7: MEAT

28. How many times a week do you eat steak, roast beef, pork chops, veal, lamb, steak sandwiches or other red meat?

Seven or more	-4
Four to six	-3
Three to four	-2
One to two	-1
Less than one	0
I don't eat red meat	+3

points: _____

29. How many times a week do you eat processed meats (corned beef, hot dogs, sausage, salami, pastrami, hoagie sandwiches, bacon, hamburgers, luncheon meats, etc.

Seven or more	-4
Four to six	-3
Three to four	-2
One to two	-1
Less than one	0
I don't eat processed meats	+3

points: _____

30. When preparing red meat, do you trim off all the visible fat before you cook it (beef, pork, lamb, veal, etc.)?

| No | -3 |

Yes   0
I don't eat red meat   +3

                        points: _____

31. When eating meat in a restaurant, do you trim away
    all the visible fat before you eat it?
                 No   –3
                 Yes   0
                 I don't eat red meat   +3

                        points: _____

                 Total points for Part 7: _____

PART 8: FAST FOOD, JUNK
FOOD, DESSERTS
32. How many times a week do you eat cookies, candy,
    cheesecake, custard pudding, ice cream, fruit pies,
    cream pies, doughnuts or other pastries, or junk foods?

Ten or more   –4
Seven to nine   –3
Three to six   –2
One to two   –1
Less than one   0
I don't eat these foods   +3

                        points: _____

33. How many times a week do you eat hamburgers, fish
    sandwiches, fried chicken, tacos, burritos, French
    fries, pizza, onion rings, etc., at fast-food restaurants,
    hamburger or pizza places?

Five or more   –4
One to four   –3
Less than one   –1
I don't eat these foods   +3

                        points: _____

34. How many times a week do you eat meals consisting mostly of canned and/or processed foods?

Seven or more	–3
Four to six	–1
One to three	–1
Less than one	0
None	+2

points: _____

Total points for Part 8: _____

PART 9: BEVERAGES

35. Which beverage do you usually drink? (Circle all that apply and average.)

Soda, coffee, tea	–3
Canned fruit juice	–2
Diet soda	–1
Water or fresh squeezed orange juice	+3

36. How many 8-oz. glasses of water do you drink a day?

None	–2
One to three	+1
Four to six	+2
Seven or more	+3

37. How many cups of coffee, tea, cocoa, cola, chocolate or other caffeine-containing liquids do you drink a day?

Four or more	–4
Three	–3
Two	–2
One	–1
I don't drink coffee or other caffeine-containing liquids	+3

points: _____

38. What kind of coffee do you drink?

Regular	–3
Decaf	–1
I don't drink coffee	+3

39. What kind of milk do you usually drink?

Whole milk (regular)	–3
Low-fat milk	–2
I don't drink milk	0
Nonfat milk (skim)	+4

points: _____

40. How many times a day do you drink skim (nonfat) milk?

None	0
One to two	+1
Three	+2
Four or more	+3

points: _____

Total points for Part 9: _____

PART 10: TOPPINGS

41. What condiments do you generally use? (Circle all that apply and average.)

Salt, sea salt or soy sauce	–3
Mustard, catsup	–2
Herbs, spices, lemon juice	+2
Garlic	+3

points: _____

42. Do you use butter or margarine on bread, vegetables or other food?

Most always	–3
Seldom	0
Never	+3

points: _____

43. Do you eat foods with gravy, mayonnaise, lard, dressing or other fatty or sugary sauces?

Most always	–3
Seldom	0
Never	+3

points: _____

Total points for Part 10: _____

PART 11: GENERAL
44. Do you eat bacon, eggs and/or sausage for breakfast?

Yes	–3
No	0

points: _____

45. Do you eat toast with butter, jelly or jam, and/or a doughnut, croissant or other pastry for breakfast?

Yes	–2
No	0

points: _____

46. Do you eat fresh fruit, whole grains and/or whole-grain cereals for breakfast?

No	0
Yes	+3

points: _____

47. What do you usually have for dessert? (Circle all that apply and average.):

Ice cream, cake, pie or pastry	–3
Ice milk	–2
Sweetened yogurt	–1
I don't eat dessert	0
Plain, nonfat yogurt	+1
Fresh fruit	+2

points: _____

48. What do you generally eat for a snack? (Circle all that apply and average.)

Pastries, candy, granola bars or cookies	–3
Chips, granola	–2
Sweetened yogurt	–1
Nothing	0
Unsweetened, nonfat yogurt	+2
Fruits, vegetables, whole-wheat bread, whole grains	+3

points: _____

49. What kind of sandwiches do you eat? (Circle all that apply and average)

Hot dogs, hamburgers, luncheon and/or packaged meats	–3
Peanut butter and/or jelly, cheese, cream cheese	–2
I don't eat sandwiches	0
Turkey, chicken or tuna (water packed)	+2
Sprouts, vegetables	+3

points: _____

50. When you eat a salad, does it contain (Circle all that apply and average.):

Mayonnaise-laden potato salad, pasta salad, cole slaw or other "salads"	−2
Pickled or canned vegetables	−2
I don't eat salads	0
Lettuce and a few slices of cucumber and tomato	+1
Four or more different fresh vegetables and/or fruits	+2
Seven or more different fresh vegetables and/or fruits	+3

points: _____

51. What do you add to your salads? (Circle all that apply and average.)

Thousand Island, French, Roquefort or Italian dressing, cheese sauce	−3
Vinegar and oil	−2
I don't eat salads	0
Raisins or small amounts of nuts or seeds	+1
Nothing, vinegar, lemon juice, vegetable or fruit juice	+3

points: _____

52. How many times a week do you eat prepared soups (canned or packaged?)

Five or more	−3
Three to four	−2
One to two	−1
None	0

points: _____

53. How many times a week do you eat salted nuts, potato chips, pretzels or other salted snacks?

Seven or more   –3
Four to six   –2
One to three   –1
None   0

points: _____

54. How many times a week do you have white-flour pancakes, waffles or sugary cereals?

Seven or more   –4
Five to six   –3
Three to four   –2
One to two   –1
None   0

points: _____

55. How many times a week do you eat deep-fried foods such as deep-fried chicken, fish or vegetables, French fries, potato chips or corn chips?

Seven or more   –5
Four to six   –4
Two to three   –3
One   –2
Never   +3

points: _____

Total points for Part 11: _____

PART 12: ALCOHOL,
SMOKING AND DRUGS
56. I drink alcoholic beverages (1 1/2 oz. liquor, 5 oz. wine, 12 oz. beer):

Four times a day   –4

Three times a day   –3
Two times a day   –2
Once a day   –1
Less than once a day   0
I don't drink alcoholic beverages   +2

points: _____

57. Do you take diuretics (medicines to lose water.)?
Yes   –2
No   0

points: _____

58. Do you take antibiotics for infections more than once
    a year?
Yes   –2
No   0

points: _____

59. Do you use laxatives?
Four to seven times a week   –3
One to three times a week   –2
I don't use laxatives   0

points: _____

60. Do you use antacids?
Regularly   –3
Occasionally   –1
Rarely or never   0

points: _____

61. (For women) Do you take birth control pills?

Yes   –3
No   0

points: _____

62. Are you taking drug therapy for high blood pressure,
arthritis, convulsions or diabetes?

Yes   –3
No   +3

points: _____

63. Do you use drugs (illicit drugs such as marijuana or
cocaine.)?

Yes   –3
No   +3

points: _____

64. Do you smoke tobacco?

Yes   –3
No   +3

points: _____

65. Do you spend more than a half hour a day in rooms
where people are smoking?

Daily   –2
Once a week or more   –1
Rarely or never   +3

points: _____

66. Do you live or work in an environment with polluted air?

Yes   –3
No   +3

points: _____

Total points for Part 12: _____

You may have wondered about some of the questions in this quiz. What, for example, does taking antacids have to do with nutrition? Quite a bit, it turns out. Many common drugs lower our levels of vitamins or minerals by making it more difficult for our bodies to absorb the nutrients from our diet. Other drugs increase our excretion of nutrients. Cigarette smoke and pollution also affect our nutritional status.

Your Grand Total Is:

Add your points from each section to get your grand total.

Part 1: _____
Part 2: _____
Part 3: _____
Part 4: _____
Part 5: _____
Part 6: _____
Part 7: _____
Part 8: _____
Part 9: _____
Part 10: _____
Part 11: _____
Part 12: _____

Grand Total: _____

What Does My Score Mean?

Again, I treat this, or any other test I give my patients, as part of the complete package of information to be gathered. Additional questions to clarify or expand upon certain areas may be necessary. Along with the complete medical history, physical examination, laboratory tests and other studies, this quiz is a valuable tool for evaluating a person.

Generally speaking, scores below -70 are good cause for concern. Your "doctor within" is staggering. I tell my patients who score -70 or below to go right home and empty their refrigerator and cupboards, then go to the market and buy a shopping basket full of Super Foods and healthy foods. Their "doctor within" needs as much help as possible to repair the damage done by the Standard American Diet.

I see a lot of scores between -1 and -69. People in this category are eating the S.A.D., with its excess fat, sugar, salt, cholesterol, additives and caffeine. With this kind of diet you may find yourself standing on the SIGNS or SYMPTOMS rungs of the HEALTH LADDER. I tell my patients in this category to eliminate the unhealthy foods from their diet and replace them with plenty of Super Foods and other healthy foods.

Scores between 0 and 59 suggest that you're eating a fairly good diet. I have my patients who score in this range study their nutritional survey carefully to see which Super Foods and other healthy foods can be added to their diet and which processed foods, canned foods, fast foods, sugary foods or fatty foods can be eliminated.

Scoring 60 or more on this nutrition quiz is an indication that you're working hand in-hand with your "doctor within," providing him the nutritional tools needed to help build health, happiness and longevity. The test may, however, indicate some ways you can improve your nutritional status.

It's true that low scores may be cause for concern, but remember that this is a learning quiz. And there's nothing to stop you from changing your eating habits and taking the quiz again. Identifying the problem, which you've done, is the first part of the solution. The second part is to make the appropriate changes. Reread Chapter Two, "Super Foods," then go back to your nutrition survey. Look at all those fatty, sugary, cholesterol-laden, additive-stuffed foods you're eating. Banish those from your diet. Replace them with Super Foods and other healthy foods that will help your "doctor within" help you.

What you do and do not eat, whether you smoke, take medicines or drugs, or live in a polluted environment, and many other factors affect your total nutritional status. Nutrition, in turn, plays an important role in the health of your "doctor within." I consider nutrition to be of prime importance, although not the only ingredient necessary for the development and maintenance of good health.

The outlook-on-life, exercise and nutrition quizzes have helped you examine yourself and your health habits. Now let's move on to laboratory tests that measure different indicators of immune system strength.

Immuno-Nutrition Laboratory Tests

After I've completed a patient's physical examination, personal and medical history, and various tests and questions, I may conduct special laboratory tests that look at the immune system. I have a regular panel of blood tests, which are routinely performed on new patients. Some of the items from the standard panel provide information on the immune system. Should I suspect an immune system problem, I may order additional tests.

Here is a list of the immune system tests I may request performed on a patient. These are not the only tests of immune-system function, but they give me an idea of what's happening inside the body. *Before I go on, let me emphasize that you shouldn't diagnose yourself as having (or not having) a certain disease based on these tests, or by comparing your results to the levels I prefer to see in my patients. Laboratory tests are only one of the diagnostic tools a physician uses: by themselves the tests may be misleading.*

But I like all my patients to know what's happening inside their bodies, to see and keep copies of their lab results and to-follow changes in these tests over time. I feel that the more you know about your health, the more likely you are to take care of yourself.

Make a photocopy of the list of tests that follows, and take it to your doctor. Tell him or her to look in your chart and give you the results of the tests that have been performed on you. Don't accept "normal" or "good" or "high" for an answer: ask for the numbers. If your doctor doesn't have these test on record, you may wish to discuss having one or more tests performed, if an immune-system problem is suspected.

The first four tests listed are simple measurements your doctor can take in the office. The rest are blood tests. In general, they are used to gauge immune-system strength and functioning, and to identify possible immune-system shortcomings. To learn what the various tests measure, see "Understanding Immune-System Tests" (Chapter Eleven).

I've indicated the levels I like to see under "My Preferred Range."

Test	Your Results	My Preferred Range
Height	_____	
Weight	_____	not obese
Triceps skin fat fold (TSF)	_____	see p. 319
Mid-arm Muscle Circumference (MAMC)	_____	see p. 320
WBC (White blood cell count)	_____	5,000-10,000
Total Lymphocyte Count	_____	2,500 or more
T-Cell count	_____	75% of lymphocytes
B-cell count	_____	25% of lymphocytes

T4/T8 Ratio	————	about 1.8/1
Total T4 cells as a %	————	35-55%
Absolute T4 count	————	385-2090
Total T8 cells as a %	————	15-39%
Absolute T8 count	————	165-1290
Immunoglobulin		
IgA	————	76-390mg/dl
IgG	————	600-1,600 mg/dl
IgM	————	40-345 mg/dl
Complement (C3)	————	80-155 mg/dl
Vitamin A	————	200-300 IU/100cc
Beta carotene	————	250-300 mcg/dl
Vitamin B_1	————	5-15+ mcg/dl
Vitamin B_2	————	4-5+ mcg/dl
Vitamin B_3	————	4-5+ mcg/dl
Vitamin B_6	————	5-25+ mg/dl
Vitamin B_{12}	————	500-1,000+ mg/dl
Folic acid	————	10-20+ mg/dl
Vitamin C	————	1.5-2.5 mg/dl
Vitamin E	————	1-2 mg/dl
Iron	————	about 100 mcg/dl
Zinc	————	about 100 mcg/dl
Cholesterol	————	100 plus age
HDL	————	50 plus
LDL	————	less than 100
CADRIF 1	————	less than 4
CADRIF 2	————	less than 3
Triglycerides	————	less than 100
Protein:		
Retinol-binding protein	————	3.0-6.0 mg
Transferin	————	200-400 mg/dl
Serum albumin	————	4.5-5.5 gm/dl

Immunomedex   _____   1 or less = very
                                    low risk
                                    2-10 = mild risk
                                    11-20 = medium
                                    risk
                                    21-30 = high risk
                                    30 = very high
                                    risk

Self-Knowledge, Not Self-Diagnosis

Knowledge is a great thing. Self-diagnosis, however, can be dangerous. The art of diagnosing a patient is difficult and requires specialized training and experience. I've included information on immune-system tests to help you better understand your immune system and how it is measured, so that you will better be able to discuss your health plans with your physician.

In Chapter Twelve you'll learn what the tests measure. For now, however, let's look at Nutri-Prevention and the supplement programs, and learn why vitamins and minerals are so important to your "doctor within."

Chapter 8

Nutri-Prevention

As far as the medical establishment is concerned, chemotherapy the use of drugs to fight disease is an almost holy word. As a group, we doctors love to prescribe drugs. If chemotherapy led to good health it might be worthwhile, but we've been fed a bill of goods. Chemotherapy does *not* keep us healthy. If these drugs are as good as doctors claim, how come so many millions and millions of Americans are still afflicted with disease?

Chemotherapy, with its failed promises and often dangerous side effects, has not reached its full potential. It is a harsh reaction to disease that should never have occurred. And chemotherapy encourages us to neglect our health. Why take care of ourselves? All we have to do is run to a doctor and get a shot of the new wonder drug, right? It was a wise person who said that if we threw all our medicines into the ocean, we'd be better off, but the fish would be in trouble.

"Dr. Fox, you're not being fair. Lots of medicines are pretty good," a patient argued the other day. Yes, some medicines work well. We will always need medicines and surgeries for those who do become ill or injure themselves. In some cases, the risk of side effects is outweighed by the compelling need for immediate relief. Most of us, however, most of the time, would be well advised to leave drugs to the fish. Instead of relying on chemotherapy to treat disease, let's adopt a new philosophy: Nutri-Prevention.

Nutri-Prevention relies not on drugs but nutrients, such as vitamins, minerals, complex carbohydrates and amino acids (the building blocks of protein), to keep your immune system in shape. While chemotherapy makes your body the battleground that disease and drugs ravage as they struggle for dominance, Nutri- Prevention helps turn your immune system into a mighty shield against disease.

Supplements are Not a Cure-All

Before we go any further, let me make it clear that vitamin and mineral pills are not magic cures for any and every disease you may have. Vitamins and minerals are like spark plugs that help keep your body's engines (enzyme systems) running smooth and strong. Some of those engines play a role in your health and happiness. As part of Nutri-Prevention, in conjunction with a diet based on Super Foods and other healthy foods, supplements help ensure that your engines have all the spark plugs they need.

Nutri-Prevention Programs to Boost The Immune System

Although every patient has individual needs, I have found that most people fall into four general categories, requiring what I call immune-system FULFILLMENT, immune-system REJUVENATION, immune-system RESTORA-TION or immune-system REBIRTH.

When I see patients in my office, I use the extensive information I've gathered to help me decide which of my four supplement programs would be most helpful for them. Having had the opportunity to examine them and study their records, I can fine-tune the program to their specific needs.

Which Program Should You Consider?

Get your score on the Nutrition Quiz from page 224, and write it here: _____

A score above 60	= 4 points
A score above -1	= 3 points
A score above -70	= 2 points
-70 or less	= 1 point

How many points did you score for the Nutrition Quiz? _____

Get your score from the Exercise Quiz on page 202 and write it here: _____

A score above 150	= 4 points
A score above 100	= 3 points
A score above 50	= 2 points
A score below 50	= 1 point

How many points did you score for the Exercise Quiz?

_____

Get your score from the Outlook-on-Life Quiz on page 196 and write it here: _____

A score above 150	= 4 points
A score above 100	= 3 points
A score above 50	= 2 points
50 or less	= 1 point

How many points did you score for the Outlook-on-Life Quiz? _____

Now put it all together:

Nutrition Quiz points: _____
Outlook-on-Life Quiz points: _____
Exercise Quiz points: _____

Add the three to get your Grand Total: _____

A grand total of nine or more suggests that you're doing an excellent job of protecting and strengthening your "doctor within." If the physical examination, personal and medical history and other studies suggest the same, I put patients in this category on my FULFILLMENT supplement program (see page 235), tailoring it to their special needs.

Most of the grand totals I see fall between six and eight. This suggests that the patient is an average American, standing on the SIGNS or SYMPTOMS rungs of the HEALTH LADDER. Not yet dancing the disease dance, this person is sputtering along, suffering from various physical and emotional diseases and discomforts. If the other information I have gathered supports this conclusion, I put him or her on my REJUVENATION supplement program (see page 237), tailoring it to their special needs.

An alarming number of patients I have seen have grand totals between three and five. These people tend to be in poor shape. Their "doctor within" is hard pressed to keep all their systems running. If the other information I have gathered on them agrees, I put the patient on my RESTORATION supplement program (see page 239), and tailor it to their special needs.

A grand total below three is scary, suggesting that the patient is in danger of a major immune-system collapse. I urge my patients who are in this category to *immediately* make important changes in their diet, life-style and outlook on life, and begin my REBIRTH supplement program (see page 242), tailoring it to their special needs. I tell my patients to purchase the vitamins and minerals separately, or in combinations that add up to or approximate the levels for their supplement program. I explain to my patients that they should divide the supplements into two or three groups and take them throughout the day, and always *with* meals. I take half my supplements at breakfast, the rest at dinner. (If I know I'm having dinner out, I put half the supplements in a little bag and carry them with me so I'll have them handy at dinnertime.)

Remember...

The test scores by themselves aren't enough to make a diagnosis. They're just one of the tools I use in evaluating a patient. As a physician, I like to know everything that my patients are taking: medicines as well as nutritional supplements. Therefore, I suggest that everyone beginning or changing their supplement program should check first with their physician.

Fulfillment Program of Supplements

If you scored above nine or more, you're doing the right things to strengthen your "doctor within" and make yourself Immune for Life. But with the stress of everyday living, toxic pollution in our air, water and food, plus the chemicals we're exposed to during the course of the day, you have to make sure you're getting all the vitamins and minerals you need to combat disease and unhappiness. I recommend to my patients in this category a supplement program I call FULFILLMENT. Every day, FULFILL-MENT provides:

Nutrient	Amount
Beta carotene	10,000 IU
Vitamin B_1 (thiamine)	15 mg
Vitamin B_2 (riboflavin)	15 mg
Vitamin B_3 (niacin)	25 mg
Vitamin B_5 (pantothenate)	25 mg
Vitamin B_6 (pyridoxine)	25 mg
Vitamin B_{12}	25 mcgm
Biotin	300 mcgm
Choline* (as phosphatidyl choline)	50 mg
Folic Acid	400 mcgm
Inositol*	50 mg
PABA*	30 mg
Vitamin C	1,000 mg
	The vitamin C should be labeled "sustained" release or "time release."
Vitamin D	400 IU

Nutrient	Amount
Vitamin E	30 IU in the form of D-Alpha Tocopherol
Calcium**	200 mg CAUTION: If you have a tendency to form kidney stones, check with your physician before taking calcium supplements. WOMEN: Add an additional 800 mg of elemental calcium to your supplement program. Post-menopausal women should add 1,000 mg.
Magnesium	200 mg Make sure you take elemental magnesium. WOMEN: Add an additional 800 mg of magnesium to your supplement program.
Potassium	99 mg Get plenty of potassium by eating lots of vegetables and fruits. See the Potassium list (page 264).
Zinc	15 mg
Copper	1 mg
Manganese	6 mg
Chromium	100 mcgm Get the Glucose Tolerance Factor (GTF) chrominium.
Selenium	25 mcgm
For women only: Iron	Women in the menstrual years, take 18 mg iron per day. Post-menopausal women, take 10 mg iron per day.

mg = milligrams
mcgm = microgram
IU = International Units
* Choline, Inositol and PABA are unofficial members of the B family of vitamins.
** This is figured as milligrams of elemental calcium. The amount of elemental calcium varies with the type of calcium taken. For example, calcium carbonate is 40% elemental calcium. Therefore, 500 mg of calcium carbonate equals 200 mg of elemental calcium.

	Percent calcium
Calcium carbonate	40
Calcium phosphate	32
Calcium gluconate	about 10
Calcium lactate	about 10

Rejuvenation Program of Supplements

If you scored between six and eight, you're getting by, but your immune system is working overtime, trying to keep you healthy. My prescription for patients in this category includes major changes in diet, exercise and stress handling, plus the following daily program of vitamin and minerals, which I call REJUVENATION:

Nutrient	Amount
Beta carotene	10,000 IU
Vitamin A	5,000 IU
Vitamin B_1 (thiamine)	25 mg
Vitamin B_2 (riboflavin)	25 mg
Vitamin B_3 (niacin)	25 mg
Vitamin B_5 (pantothenate)	100 mg
Vitamin B_6 (pyridoxine)	50 mg
Vitamin B_{12}	50 mcgm
Biotin	300 mcgm
Choline* (as phosphatidyl choline)	100 mg
Folic Acid	400 mcgm
Inositol*	100 mg

Nutrient	Amount
PABA*	80 mg
Vitamin C	2,000 mg
	The vitamin C should be labeled "sustained" release or "time release."
Vitamin D	400 IU
Vitamin E	200 IU in the form of D-Alpha Tocopherol
Calcium**	300 mg
	CAUTION: If you have a tendency to form kidney stones, check with your physician before taking calcium supplements. WOMEN: Add an additional 700 mg of elemental calcium to your supplement program. Post-menopausal women should add 1,000 mg.
Magnesium	300 mg
	Make sure you take elemental magnesium. WOMEN: Add an additional 700 mg of elemental magnesium to your supplement program.
Potassium	99 mg
	Get plenty of potassium by eating lots of vegetables and fruits. See the Potassium list (page 264)
Zinc	30 mg
Copper	2 mg
Manganese	6 mg
Chromium	100 mcgm
	Get the Glucose Tolerance Factor (GTF) chromium.
Selenium	50 mcgm

Nutrient	Amount
For women only: Iron	Women in the menstrual years, take 18 mg iron per day. Post-menopausal women, take 10 mg iron per day.

mg = milligrams
mcgm = microgram
IU = International Units
* Choline, Inositol and PABA are unofficial members of the B family of vitamins.
** This is figured as milligrams of elemental calcium. The amount of elemental calcium varies with the type of calcium taken. For example, calcium carbonate is 40% elemental calcium. Therefore, 500 mg of calcium carbonate equals 200 mg of elemental calcium.

	Percent calcium
Calcium carbonate	40
Calcium phosphate	32
Calcium gluconate	about 10
Calcium lactate	about 10

Along with the vitamin and minerals supplements in the REJUVENATION program, I suggest my patients take:

DLPA	750 mg	Once a day, taken with breakfast.

DLPA stands for di-phenylalanine. Phenylalanine is one of the essential amino acids your body uses to manufacture proteins. See page 245 to learn more about DLPA.

Restoration Program of Supplements

If, by virtue of your test scores, you find yourself in the RESTORATION category, your diet, exercise habits and/ or outlook on life are poor. You're probably eating a lot of fatty, sugary, processed, cholesterol- and additive-laden foods. You exercise sporadically, if at all. It's likely that you're unhappy and view the world as a depressing place.

Patients I have seen in this category tend to be standing on the SYMPTOMS or MEASURABLE ILLNESS rungs of the HEALTH LADDER. Their medical files are often voluminous, and they've been to many doctors in search of a cure for their recurrent physical and emotional problems.

Unless the trend is reversed, their "doctor within" will soon be too weak to protect their health. I urge my patients in this category to start on the daily RESTO-RATION supplement program ASAP.

Nutrient	Amount
Beta carotene	15,000 IU
Vitamin A (retinol)	7,500 IU
Vitamin B$_1$ (thiamine)	50 mg
Vitamin B$_2$ (riboflavin)	50 mg
Vitamin B$_3$ (niacin)	50 mg
Vitamin B$_5$ (pantothenate)	150 mg
Vitamin B$_6$ (pyridoxine)	100 mg
Vitamin B$_{12}$	100 mcgm
Biotin	300 mcgm
Choline* (as phosphatidyl choline)	200 mg
Folic acid	400 mcgm
Inositol*	200 mg
PABA*	100 mg
Vitamin C	3,000 mg The vitamin C should be labeled "sustained release" or "time release."
Vitamin D	400 IU
Vitamin E	300 IU in the form of D-Alpha Tocopherol
Calcium**	400 mg CAUTION: If you have a tendency to form kidney stones,

Nutrient	Amount
	check with your physician before taking calcium supplements. WOMEN: Add an additional 600 mg of elemental calcium to your supplement program. Post-menopausal women should add 1,000 mg.
Magnesium	400 mg Make sure you are taking elemental magnesium. WOMEN: Add an additional 600 mg of magnesium to your supplement program.
Potassium	99 mg Get plenty of potassium by eating lots of vegetables and fruits. See the Potassium list (page 264).
Zinc	50 mg
Copper	2 mg
Manganese	10 mg
Chromium	150 mcgm Get the Glucose Tolerance Factor (GTF) chromium.
Selenium	100 mcgm
For women only: Iron	Women in the menstrual years, take 18 mg iron per day. Post-menopausal women, take 10 mg iron per day.

mg = milligrams
mcgm = microgram
IU = International Units
* Choline, Inositol and PABA are unofficial members of the B family of vitamins.
** This is figured as milligrams of elemental calcium. The amount of elemental

calcium varies with the type of calcium taken. For example, calcium carbonate is 40% elemental calcium. Therefore, 500 mg of calcium carbonate equals 200 mg of elemental calcium.

	Percent calcium
Calcium carbonate	40
Calcium phosphate	32
Calcium gluconate	about 10
Calcium lactate	about 10

To complete the RESTORATION add:

DLPA	750 mg	Twice a day, one capsule with breakfast, and one with lunch

DLPA stands for di-phenylalanine. Phenylalanine is one of the essential amino acids your body uses to manufacture proteins. See page 197 to learn more about DLPA.

Rebirth Program of Supplements

Patients I see in this category tend to be the sickest and/ or the most stressed. They seem headed on a collision course with trouble if they aren't already in the hospital with a serious disease. These people are standing on the MEASURABLE ILLNESS or CHRONIC ILLNESS rungs of the HEALTH LADDER. But it's never too late to try and push them back up to the VIBRANT HEALTH rung by making major changes in life-style, diet and exercise habits to bolster their "doctor within." This is the daily supplement program I recommend to my patients in the REBIRTH category:

Nutrient	Amount
Beta carotene	20,000 IU
Vitamin A	10,000 IU
Vitamin B$_1$ (thiamine)	100 mg
Vitamin B$_2$ (riboflavin)	100 mg

Nutrient	Amount
Vitamin B$_3$ (niacin)	100 mg
Vitamin B$_5$ (pantothenate)	200 mg
Vitamin B$_6$ (pyridoxine)	200 mg
Vitamin B$_{12}$	200 mcgm
Biotin	300 mcgm
Choline* (as phosphatidylcholine)	300 mg
Folic Acid	800 mcgm
Inositol*	300 mg
PABA*	200 mg
Vitamin C	4,000 mg
	The vitamin C should be labeled "sustained release" or "time release."
Vitamin D	400 IU
Vitamin E	400 IU
	in the form of D-Alpha Tocopherol
Calcium**	500 mg
	CAUTION: If you have a tendency to form kidney stones, check with your physician before taking calcium supplements. WOMEN: Add an additional 500 mg of elemental calcium to your supplement program. Post-menopausal women should add 1000 mg.
Magnesium	500 mg
	Make sure you take elemental magnesium. WOMEN: Add an additional 500 mg of magnesium to your supplement program.
Potassium	99 mg
	Get plenty of potassium by eating lots of vegetables and

Nutrient	Amount
	fruits. See the Potassium list (page 264)
Zinc	50 mg
Copper	2 mg
Manganese	10 mg
Chromium	200 mcgm Get the Glucose Tolerance Factor (GTF) chromium.
Selenium	200 mcgm
For women only: Iron	Women in the premenstrual years, take 18 mg iron per day. Post-menopausal women, take 10 mg iron per day.

mg = milligrams
mcgm = microgram
IU = International Units
* Choline, Inositol and PABA are unofficial members of the B family of vitamins.
** This is figured as milligrams of elemental calcium. The amount of elemental calcium varies with the type of calcium taken. For example, calcium carbonate is 40% elemental calcium. Therefore, 500 mg of calcium carbonate equals 200 mg of elemental calcium.

	Percent calcium
Calcium carbonate	40
Calcium phosphate	32
Calcium gluconate	about 10
Calcium lactate	about 10

To complete the "Rebirth" add:

DLPA	750 mg	Three times a day: one capsule with breakfast, one with lunch and one with dinner.

DLPA stands for di-phenylalanine. Phenylalanine is one of the essential amino acids your body uses to manufacture proteins. To learn more about DLPA, keep reading, and see footnote below for an important warning.

DLPA, the Endorphins and Your Immune System

DLPA* is included in three of the four Nutri-Prevention plans because it's a natural, safe and effective tool for energizing your immune system. As Barry and I explained in our book, *DLPA to End Chronic Pain and Depression,* DLPA can relieve the pain of arthritis, low back pain, whiplash and even the pain of cancer. Available at vitamin and health food stores across the country, it's a natural substance the body needs, and it's found in many foods. DLPA works by protecting and enhancing the endorphins in your body. The endorphins actually block pain signals from reaching the higher centers in your brain, and lift your mood. New studies have shown that the endorphins also strengthen the immune system. That's why DLPA is part of my Nutri-Prevention program.

What Vitamins and Minerals Can Do for You

People are confused by the profusion of information about vitamin and mineral supplements. What do vitamins and minerals do? Why should I take them? Here's a brief description of the valuable roles played by vitamins and some minerals. This will help you understand why certain vitamins and minerals are included in the four supplement programs of Nutri-Prevention. For more information on the relationship between vitamins and minerals and your immune system, see Chapter 10.

* I recommend against using DLPA during pregnancy or lactation. Pregnant or lactating women should not expose the fetus to anything other than their normal diet. Neither should persons suffering from the genetic disease phenylketonuria (PKU) take DLPA—they cannot metabolize phenylalanine normally. This also applies to those on phenylalanine-restricted diets. Neither do I recommend the use of DLPA for children under age 14. As an Internist and Cardiologist, I do not usually treat children. However, children's physician's may wish to examine the DLPA literature.

VITAMINS
VITAMIN A

Functions: the single most important vitamin with respect to the immune system • necessary for night vision and protein synthesis • promotes fertility • stimulates bone growth • assists in growth and repair of body cells • essential for healthy skin and respiratory tract, as well as the linings of esophagus, stomach, intestine, colon, rectum, gall bladder, kidneys and urinary tract • prompts secretion of digestive "juices" • necessary for growth in the young.

Deficiency signs and symptoms: increased susceptibility to infection • night blindness and other eye problems • dryness, thickness and eruptions of the skin • dry, brittle nails • softness of bones and teeth.

Vitamin A's enemies: mineral oil • alcohol • light • high temperature • air.

VITAMIN B_1 (thiamine)

Functions: vital for a healthy immune system • necessary for the conversion of carbohydrates into energy in the nervous system and in muscles.

Deficiency signs and symptoms: mental problems such as loss of mental alertness, irritability, memory loss, confusion and depression • fatigue • loss of appetite • heart irregularities • numbness, tingling and weakness in the extremities and other parts of body (polyneuritis) • constipation • tenderness in the calves • burning sensations in the feet • the classic B_1 deficiency disease is beriberi • extreme deficiency leads to heart failure, degeneration of nerve endings, and death.

Vitamin B_1's enemies: heat • air • excessive cooking of food • caffeine • alcohol • excessive dietary sugar.

VITAMIN B$_2$ (riboflavin)

Functions: vital for a healthy immune system • plays a role in the metabolism (usage) of fats, carbohydrates and protein, as well as cell respiration and growth • necessary for the manufacture and repair of body tissues.

Deficiency signs and symptoms: dizziness • trembling • insomnia • lassitude • cracks and sores in the corner of the mouth • redness of the mouth and palate • sore, red tongue • poor growth of hair, nails and skin • oily skin • eye problems including inflammation of the whites of the eyes, cloudiness of the cornea, unusual sensitivity to light, a burning sensation, a "gritty" feeling under the eyelids • dermatitis of the scrotum.

Vitamin B$_2$'s enemies: light • excessive boiling of food • stress • excess dietary sugar • alcohol.

VITAMIN B$_3$ (niacin)

Functions: vital for health and maintenance of skin, mouth, intestines and nerves • necessary for the extraction of energy from carbohydrates, fat and protein • crucial for the conversion of the amino acid tryptophan into a neurotransmitter.

Deficiency signs and symptoms: headaches • irritability • insomnia • fatigue • muscle weakness • loss of appetite, nausea and vomiting • diarrhea • skin eruptions • skin problems, such as dryness and scales • canker sores • the classic deficiency disease is pellagra, with symptoms of diarrhea, dermatitis, dementia and, in extreme cases, death.

Vitamin B$_3$'s enemies: excessive boiling of food • alcohol.

VITAMIN B₅ (pantothenic acid)

Functions: vital for a healthy immune system • important in metabolism (use) of protein, fat and carbohydrate • necessary for the manufacture of antibodies • plays role in maintaining health of nervous system.

Deficiency signs and symptoms: decreased resistance to disease • depression • irritability • fatigue • headaches • dizziness • lack of coordination • weakness • malaise • insomnia • tremors • sweating • weakness • muscle soreness • irregular heart rhythms • dermatitis. It is very difficult to suffer from a deficiency of vitamin B5 because it's found in so many foods. But due to the stresses of modern living, we need generous amounts of this vitamin.

Vitamin B₅'s enemies: cooking • processing and canning of foods • caffeine • alcohol • excessive boiling of food • deep freezing and thawing.

VITAMIN B₆ (pyridoxine)

Functions: second only to vitamin A with respect to importance for immune system function • essential for proper function of the nervous system • necessary for proper absorption of vitamin B₁₂, and for formation of red blood cells • part of the enzyme that converts glycogen (energy stored in the liver) into glucose • necessary for the manufacture and proper action of DNA and RNA • important for the conversion of the amino acid tryptophan to the neurotransmitter serotonin.

Deficiency signs and symptoms: immune-system problems • depression • nervousness • irritability • insomnia • loss of appetite • weight loss • weakness • smoothness of tongue and soreness of mouth • cracks in the skin on the sides of the mouth • pains, numbness and tingling of the extremities • abnormal heart rhythms.

Vitamin B_6's enemies: heat • excessive boiling of food • excess dietary sugar • alcohol.

WARNING: B_6 should not be taken with the anti-Parkinson disease drug, L-Dopa. Taken in very large doses, 2,000 to 6,000 mg per day, it can cause a neuritis. Persons on the antitubercular drug, INH, however, *should* be taking B_6 supplements.

VITAMIN B_{12}

Functions: vital for a healthy immune system • needed for production and growth of red blood cells in the bone marrow and their release into circulation when mature • necessary for DNA synthesis • plays a role in maintaining the myelin sheath that protects nerve cells.

Deficiency signs and symptoms: a reduction in red blood cell, white blood cell, and platelet counts, which can cause anemia and immune system problems • irritability • headaches • forgetfulness • dizziness • fatigue • weakness • heart palpitations • enlarged spleen • numbness and tingling of the extremities • sore tongue • constipation • loss of appetite • the classic vitamin B12 deficiency disease of pernicious anemia.

Vitamin B_{12}'s enemies: excessive boiling of food • sunlight • alcohol.

BIOTIN
Biotin is a member of the B family of vitamins.

Functions: vital for a healthy immune system • involved in a wide variety of metabolic reactions in the body • necessary for maintenance of healthy skin, hair, nerves, bone marrow and sex glands • plays a role in extracting energy from carbohydrates, fat and protein.

Deficiency signs and symptoms: depression • skin

inflammations • nausea and loss of appetite • vomiting • chest and muscle pain • increased cholesterol levels • blood sugar irregularities • deficiencies in the manufacture of protein • extreme exhaustion • hair loss • dermatitis • paleness and smoothness of the tongue.

Biotin's enemies: alcohol • food processing • excessive boiling of food.

CHOLINE
Choline is an unofficial member of the B family of vitamins. Because it can be synthesized in the liver, it is not regarded as a true vitamin.

Functions: associated with the utilization of fat and cholesterol • important for the maintenance and health of the nerve cover (myelin) • essential for transmission of nerve impulses • necessary for the formation of lecithin and the production of acetylcholine, (a neurotransmitter) • helps prevent accumulation of fats in the liver and other organs.

Deficiency signs and symptoms: liver problems and hardening of the arteries • choline deficiency may be a factor in Alzheimer's disease, nerve degeneration, elevated blood pressure and cholesterol, stroke and immune-system problems.

Choline's enemies: food processing • excessive boiling of food • alcohol.

FOLIC ACID
Folic acid is a member of the B family of vitamins.

Functions: vital for a healthy immune system • important for metabolism of RNA and DNA, protein synthesis and formation or red blood cells • many of folic acid's functions are associated with vitamin B_{12}.

Deficiency signs and symptoms: irritability • forgetfulness • dementia • mental retardation • anemia •
inflammation of nerves • spinal cord damage • loss of energy
• loss of appetite and weight • diarrhea • vomiting •
indigestion • sore mouth and tongue • weakness • cervical
abnormalities • poor growth in children • congenital
malformations in babies.

Folic Acid's enemies: excessive boiling of food • food
processing • heat • alcohol.

INOSITOL
Inositol is an unofficial member of the B family of vitamins.
It is not generally regarded as a true vitamin because it
can be manufactured in the body.

Functions: important for nourishment of the brain •
helps prevent build-up of fats in liver and other organs
• has mild anti-anxiety effects • helps control blood-
cholesterol levels • helps maintain healthy hair.

Deficiency signs and symptoms: insufficient data
available. Inositol's enemies: excessive boiling of food •
food processing • alcohol • coffee.

PABA (para aminobenzoic acid)
PABA is an unofficial member of the B family of vitamins.
It not considered a true vitamin for humans.

Functions: has a certain value as an antioxidant (protects
cells against damage caused by inappropriate combining
with oxygen).

Deficiency signs and symptoms: deficiency in animals
can lead to anemia, as well as premature graying of the
hair.

PABA's enemies: excessive boiling of food • food
processing • alcohol.

VITAMIN C

Functions: vital for a healthy immune system • helps protect body cells from oxidation (damage due to inappropriate combining of molecules with oxygen) • plays a vital role in forming collagen, the substance that holds the body's cells together • encourages iron absorption • functions in regulation of cholesterol levels • necessary for proper functioning of the brain and nerves • important for health of capillaries and sex organs.

Deficiency signs and symptoms: lassitude • weakness • irritability • vague muscle and joint pains • loss of weight • inflamed and bleeding gums • loosening of the teeth • hemorrhages under the skin • bruising • the classic vitamin C deficiency disease of scurvy.

Vitamin C's enemies: cigarettes • heat • excessive boiling of food • light • stress.

VITAMIN D

Functions: promotes absorption of calcium and phosphate.

Deficiency signs and symptoms: nervous-system disorders • tooth decay • the classic vitamin D deficiency diseases are rickets (in children), osteomalacia (in adults) and osteoporosis (thinning of the bone).

Vitamin D's enemies: anything that reduces the amount of sunlight you receive (such as smog and staying indoors all the time) interferes with vitamin D production by your body.

VITAMIN E (tocopherol)

Functions: vital for a healthy immune system • protects body cells against oxidation • helps control free radicals (unstable molecules in the body that can cause cancer and other problems).

Deficiency signs and symptoms: nervous-system disorders • gastrointestinal problems • premature aging of the skin • dry, itchy skin • infertility • destruction of red blood cells in infants, leading to anemia.

Vitamin E's enemies: mineral oil • cooking and processing of foods • heat • freezing • iron • chlorine.

MINERALS
CALCIUM

Functions: necessary for bone formation • helps blood coagulate • plays a role in activating certain enzymes • assists in regulating capillary and cell permeability • important for nerve-impulse transmission and muscle contractions.

Deficiency signs and symptoms: rickets (in children) • osteomalacia (in adults) • osteoporosis (thinning of bones) • joint pains • muscle cramps • heart palpitations • insomnia • cramping of muscles • nervousness and irritability • numbness and tingling of extremities • tooth decay.
Calcium's enemies: chronic stress • alcohol • high protein diets.

CHLORIDE

Functions: necessary for maintaining the body's acid-base balance • essential for stomach acid • helps preserve body fluids.

Deficiency signs and symptoms: fatigue • weakness • heart irregularities • cramping of the muscles.

Chloride's enemies: fad diets and starvation diets.

CHROMIUM

Functions: part of the glucose tolerance factor (GTF) and, as such, helps maintain a normal blood sugar level • helps regulate cholesterol and triglyceride (fat) levels.

Deficiency signs and symptoms: abnormalities in the body's handling of glucose, which can lead to diabetes • arteriosclerosis and cardiovascular disease.

Chromium's enemies: excessive boiling of food • refining of foods.

COPPER

Functions: vital for a healthy immune system • necessary for normal development of bone, connective tissue and the central nervous system • vital for production of RNA • assists in absorption of iron • works with vitamin C in forming elastin (part of the elastic muscle fibers) • plays a role in the manufacture of myelin (the fatty sheath that surrounds and protects nerve fibers) • involved with the birth of red blood cells and hemoglobin • necessary for cardiovascular integrity.

Deficiency signs and symptoms: an anemia and its associated symptoms (fatigue, weakness, shortness of breath).

Copper's enemies: excess dietary zinc.

IRON

Functions: vital for a healthy immune system • part of the hemoglobin molecule that binds oxygen in the red blood cells.

Deficiency signs and symptoms: weakness and fatigue.

Iron's enemies: lack of stomach acid • extreme diets in which only or mostly green vegetables are eaten • intestinal diseases which speed transit of food through intestines • poor absorption of dietary fat (leading to excess fat in intestine interfering with iron absorption).

MAGNESIUM

Functions: vital for a healthy immune system • involved with energy formation and transfer, carbohydrate metabolism, manufacture of protein, proper nutrition of the heart and neuromuscular transmission.

Deficiency signs and symptoms: personality changes • fatigue • muscle weakness • heart irregularities • muscle spasms.

Magnesium's enemies: prolonged fasting • persistent vomiting • chronic diarrhea • surgery • severe burns • alcohol • high-protein diets.

MANGANESE

Functions: vital for a healthy immune system • important for formation of the main thyroid hormone • necessary for proper utilization of vitamins C, B_1 and biotin, and for production of acetylcholine, an important neurotransmitter.

Deficiency signs and symptoms: a deficiency in animals results in sterility in both sexes, skeletal abnormalities.

Manganese's enemies: refining of foods.

PHOSPHORUS

Functions: necessary for good bone and teeth structure and a healthy nervous system • helps stimulate muscle contractions • plays a role in extracting energy from food.

Deficiency signs and symptoms: loss of appetite • nausea • fatigue • weakness • vague and persistent bone pains.

Phosphorus' enemies: excessive ingestion of antacids.

POTASSIUM

Functions: found in all cells • necessary for cellular life.

Deficiency signs and symptoms: generalized muscle weakness and fatigue • irregular heartbeat • muscle weakness • muscle paralysis • lung failure • kidney failure.

Potassium's enemies: alcohol • coffee • diets high in refined sugar • high-protein fad diets.

SELENIUM

Functions: vital for a healthy immune system • works with vitamin E to protect against oxidation • part of the important enzyme that quenches free radicals • reduces poisonous effects of mercury, cadmium and other toxic minerals in the body.

Possible Deficiency signs and symptoms: cardiovascular disease • Sudden Infant Death (SID) • premature aging • some cases of heart failure.

Selenium's enemies: food processing • cooking.

ZINC

Functions: vital for a healthy immune system • a necessary part of over 100 enzyme ("spark plug") systems of the body • essential for the formation of insulin and protein.

Deficiency sign and symptoms: decreased growth in youngsters • failure of sexual development • decreased

mental activity • poor appetite • fatigue • skin eruptions
• poor wound healing • decreased sense of smell and/
or taste.

Zinc's enemies: alcohol • kidney disease • burns • stress.

This brief look at what I consider to be the major
vitamins and minerals only begins to scratch the surface;
volumes have been written on the individual nutrients.
But it gives you an idea of the importance of these nutrients
to your immune system and your health in general. For
more on the immune-system functions of some of the
nutrients, see Chapter Ten.

Foods Full of Nutrients

In addition to the supplements I've listed, you'll find
vitamins, minerals and other nutrients in the Super Foods
and other healthy foods I've advised you to eat. Here are
lists of foods that contain ample amounts of some of the
vitamins and minerals we've talked about. You'll notice
that most of these foods are the vegetables, fruits and whole
grains your "doctor within" loves. Starred (*) foods are
Super Foods. Double-starred foods (**) are high in fat
and/or cholesterol and should be eaten only in small
amounts.

BETA CAROTENE

Apricots
*Broccoli
Buttermilk Squash
*Cantaloupes
*Carrots
*Collards
Endives
*Kale
Mangoes
Mustard Greens
Nectarines
Papayas

*Parsley
Red Chili Peppers
Romaine Lettuce
*Scallions (Green Onions)
*Spinach
*Sweet Potatoes
*Sweet Red Peppers
Swiss Chard
Turnips
Watercress
Winter Squash

VITAMIN A

**Beef Liver	Low-Fat Cheese
**Chicken Livers	Low-Fat Milk Products
**Fish-Liver Oils	

VITAMIN B₁ (thiamine)

**Almonds	*Navy Beans
*Buckwheat	*Pinto Beans
*Garbanzo Beans	*Red Beans (Chick Peas)
*Split Peas	*Garlic
*Wild Rice	*Green Beans
*Whole-Grain Rice	**Hazelnuts
*Whole-Grain Rye	*Lentils
*Whole-Grain Oats	*Lima Beans
*Whole-Grain Wheat	*Millet

VITAMIN B₂ (riboflavin)

**Almonds	Okra
Beet Greens	*Parsley
*Black-Eyed Peas	**Pine Nuts
Brewer's Yeast	*Pinto Beans
*Broccoli	*Red Beans
Chicken	**Salmon
*Collards	**Sesame Seeds
Hot Red Peppers	*Split Peas
*Kale	Turkey
*Lentils	Wheat Bran
*Millet	Wheat Germ
Mushrooms	*Whole-Grain Rye
Mustard Greens	Wild Rice
*Navy Beans	Yogurt

VITAMIN B₃ (Niacin)

**Almonds	**Pine Nuts
*Barley	Prunes
Brewer's Yeast	Red Chili Peppers
Brook Trout	**Salmon
*Buckwheat	**Sesame Seeds
Chicken (White Meat)	**Shrimp

Dates
Haddock
Halibut
Mushrooms

*Split Peas
Turkey (White Meat)
*Whole-Grain Rice
*Whole-Grain Wheat

VITAMIN B₅ (pantothenic acid)

*Beans
Brewer's Yeast
Fish
Green Leafy Vegetables
*Lentils
**Meat

**Nuts
*Peas
Wheat Bran
Wheat Germ
*Whole-Grain Cereals

VITAMIN B₆ (pyridoxine)

Albacore
Bananas
*Barley
*Black-Eyed Peas
Brook Trout
*Brussels Sprouts
*Buckwheat
*Cantaloupes
*Cauliflower
Chestnuts
Cod
*Garbanzo Beans
  (chick peas)
Halibut
**Hazelnuts
*Kale
*Leeks
*Lentils

*Navy Beans
Perch
*Pinto Beans
Popcorn
Potatoes
*Red Cabbage
*Salmon
Sardines
*Spinach
*Sweet Potatoes
Tuna
Turnip Greens
**Walnuts
Wheat Bran
*Whole-Grain Rice
*Whole-Grain Rye
*Whole-Grain Wheat
*Lima Beans

VITAMIN B₁₂

Brook Trout
**Cheese
**Eggs
Flounder
Haddock

Perch
**Salmon
Sardines
Scallops
Tuna

Halibut   Yogurt
**Milk

BIOTIN

*Beans   *Lentils
**Beef Liver   **Milk
Brewer's Yeast   **Peanuts
*Brown Rice   *Peas
**Cheese   Wheat Bran
Corn   Wheat Germ
**Egg Yolks

CHOLINE

*Beans   *Lentils
Brewer's Yeast   **Liver
Chicken   **Nuts
Corn   *Peas
**Egg Yolk   Wheat Germ
Leafy Green Vegetables   Whole-Wheat Bread

FOLIC ACID

**Almonds   *Cauliflower
Apricots   Chicken Livers
Asparagus   Endives
*Beans   *Kale
**Beef Liver   Mustard Greens
Brewer's Yeast   Okra
*Broccoli   **Pecans
*Brown Rice   *Spinach
*Brussels Sprouts   Turnip Greens
*Cantaloupes   **Walnuts
*Carrots

INOSITOL

Bananas   Corn
*Beans   Grapefruits
Brewers Yeast   *Lentils
*Brown Rice   *Peas
*Cabbage   **Peanuts

*Cantaloupes
Chicken

Raisins
Wheat Germ

PABA

Brewer's Yeast
Wheat Germ

*Whole Grains

VITAMIN C

Asparagus
*Black-eyed Peas
*Broccoli
*Brussels Sprouts
*Cabbage
*Cantaloupes
*Cauliflower
*Collards
Cranberries
Grapefruits
*Green Beans
*Green Peas
Guavas
Honeydew Melon
*Kale
Lemons
*Lima Beans
Lime Juice
Mangoes

Mustard Greens
Okra
Oranges
**Oysters
*Papayas
*Parsley
Persimmons
Radishes
Raspberries
*Scallions (Green Onions)
*Spinach
Strawberries
*Sweet Red Peppers
Swiss Chard
Tangerines
Turnip Greens
Tomatoes
Yellow Summer Squash

VITAMIN D

**Fish-Liver Oil
**Herring
**Kippers
Nonfat (Skim) Milk

Nonfat Powdered Milk
**Salmon
**Sardines

VITAMIN E

*Broccoli
*Brussels Sprouts
*Green Beans
*Green Leafy Vegetables

**Nuts
*Peas
Tomatoes
Wheat Germ

**Lean Meat   **Wheat Germ Oil
**Milk   *Whole Grains

CALCIUM

**Almonds   Lemons
 Asparagus   *Lentils
*Barley   Milk, Low-Fat
 Beet Greens   *Millet
 Beets   *Onions
*Broccoli   Oranges
*Buckwheat   *Parsley
 Buttermilk   Pineapples
*Cabbage   Romaine Lettuce
*Cantaloupes   Rutabagas
*Carrots   **Sesame Seeds
*Cauliflower   *Spinach
 Celery   Strawberries
 Cherries   Summer Squash
*Collards   *Sweet Potatoes
 Cottage Cheese, low-fat   Turnip Greens
 Dandelion Greens   **Walnuts
*Garlic   Watercress
 Globe Artichokes   *Whole-Grain Rice
 Grapes   *Whole-Grain Wheat
*Green Beans   Winter Squash
*Green Peas   Yogurt

CHLORIDE

 Chicken   Kelp
**Eggs   Turkey
 Fish   *Whole Grains

NOTE: Table salt is part chloride and part sodium (sodium chloride), but I don't advocate eating salt or adding salt to your food.

CHROMIUM

 Apples   *Navy Beans
 Bananas   Oranges
 Blueberries   Parsnips

Brewer's Yeast
*Cabbage
*Carrots
Chicken
Cornmeal
Green Peppers
Mushrooms

Potatoes
*Spinach
Strawberries
Wheat Bran
Wheat Germ
Whole-Wheat Bread

COPPER

*Beans
*Lentils
**Liver

*Peas
**Oysters

IRON

**Almonds
Apricots
*Beans
Beet Greens
Dandelion Greens
*Dried Split Peas
Grapes
*Kidney Beans
Leafy Green Vegetables
*Lentils
Millet
**Oysters

*Parsley
*Peaches
**Pecans
Plums
Potatoes
**Sesame Seeds
*Spinach
Swiss Chard
**Walnuts
*Whole-Grain Oats
*Whole-Grain Wheat

MAGNESIUM

**Almonds
Apples
Asparagus
Bananas
*Barley
Beets
*Broccoli
*Cabbage
*Cantaloupes
*Carrots
Celery

Milk, Nonfat
*Millet
Mushrooms
*Onions
Oranges
*Parsley
**Pecans
Pineapples
Plums
*Spinach
Tomatoes

Chicken
*Collards
Corn
*Dry Beans
*Fresh Green Peas
*Garlic
Grapes

Turkey
**Walnuts
Winter Squash
*Whole-Grain Rice
*Whole-Grain Rye
*Whole-Grain Wheat

MANGANESE

Blueberries
Buckwheat
*Ginger
*Oat Bran
**Peanuts
Pineapples

Rice Bran
*Spinach
**Walnuts
Wheat Bran
*Whole-Grain Oats
*Whole-Grain Rice

PHOSPHORUS

Fish
**Nuts
Poultry

**Seeds
*Whole Grains

POTASSIUM

Apricots
Bananas
*Carrots
Flounder
Leafy Green Vegetables
*Lentils

Orange Juice
*Peaches
Potatoes
Skim Milk
Tomatoes
Winter Squash

SELENIUM

**Almonds
Apple Cider Vinegar
*Barley
*Cabbage
*Carrots
Chicken
Cod
*Garlic
*Green Beans

Mushrooms
*Onions
Oranges
**Pecans
Radishes
Red Swiss Chard
Scallops
**Shrimp
Turkey

**Hazelnuts
*Kidney Beans
**King Crab
Milk, Nonfat

Turnips
*Whole-Grain Oats
*Whole-Grain Rice
*Whole-Grain Wheat

ZINC

**Almonds
Black Pepper
*Buckwheat
*Carrots
Chicken
Chili Powder
Cinnamon
**Clams
Corn
Dry Mustard
Ginger Roots
*Green Peas
Haddock
*Lima Beans
**Milk

***Oysters
Paprika
**Pecans
**Sardines
*Split Peas
**Sunflower Seeds
Thyme
Tuna
Turkey
Turnips
**Walnuts
Wheat Bran
Wheat Germ
*Whole-Grain Oats
*Whole-Grain Wheat

*** Oysters from the Atlantic Ocean contain more zinc than Pacific oysters.

Supplements Do Not Replace Foods

As part of the full Immune for Life program, Nutri-Prevention can give your "doctor within" a big boost. But please, do not use vitamin and mineral supplements as a substitute for nutritious eating. Supplements are just that: something that's added to your regular regimen. The FULFILLMENT, REJUVENATION, RESTORATION and REBIRTH programs help fill nutrient gaps and add strength to your "doctor within,;' but they aren't meant to replace everyday healthy eating. Be sure to eat plenty of Super Foods and other healthy foods. In the right amounts, vitamin and mineral supplements can be extremely helpful. But too much of anything, even a good thing, can be dangerous. So please resist the temptation to double or triple your supplement levels.

I have to admit, however, that we doctors don't always agree on how much is enough. The Recommended Daily Allowance will keep you out of the hospital. How much is it necessary to take for the best possible health? The debate is raging, and slowly a consensus seems to be emerging that we could benefit from higher levels of many vitamins and minerals. I believe that in the future we will see RDAs much higher than they are now.

Nobel laureate Dr. Linus Pauling told an interesting story at the Second International Symposium on Stress Management, in 1979. Speaking to an audience of physicians and scientists, including four other Nobel prize winners, Dr. Pauling held up a glass test tube filled with white powder. He explained that the test tube contained 13 grams of vitamin C powder, the amount of vitamin C a 150-pound jackass produces every day. Then he held up a second test tube that was empty. This, he said, represents the amount of vitamin C a human makes every day: none. Next he showed a third test tube, containing a tiny bit of powder. This is how much vitamin C the government says we need every day, he said.

He looked from one test tube to the next, comparing the amount of vitamin C a jackass makes to the amount the government says humans need. Then, to the great delight of the audience, he smiled and said: "Wouldn't you know it? A jackass knows more about vitamin C than our government does."

It's too bad we humans aren't like jackasses, and just about every other animal. They can make their own vitamin C; we can't. Our bodies don't manufacture any vitamins and minerals in sufficient amounts. We're at the mercy of our diet to provide these vital substances. So make sure that everything you eat has lots of the vitamins, minerals, complex carbohydrates, fiber and other nutrients you need to build vibrant health and happiness.

Part 3

Immune for Life Information File

Chapter 9

Your Immune System

*R*emember those kaleidoscopes we enjoyed looking into so much as children? Wasn't it marvelous, the infinite variety of patterns produced by simply turning one end of the tube? Well, kaleidoscopes contain but a few pieces of colored glass, yet they manage to produce an incredible number of visual patterns. In some respects your immune system is like a kaleidoscope. With a limited number of weapons, it puts up an almost endless variety of defenses against disease.

Because there are so many kinds of disease eager to challenge your defense network, your immune system has developed a variety of immune "soldiers," each with its own weapons and method of attack. Some parts of your immune system don't actually engage in battle. Instead, they act like computers, storing information on the enemy and its characteristics, or serve to control other immune cells.

The individual parts of the immune system are powerful, each in their own way. No single component of the immune system, however, is a match for the many diseases that are eager to harm you. But taken as a whole, the immune system packs an incredible wallop, each part contributing in its own special way.

And a lot of parts there are. You may have heard these terms tossed about: T-cells, B-cells, killer cells, interferon, lymphocytes, phagocytes, T4, lymph glands, and so on. Let's begin this brief discussion of the immune system by looking at the white blood cells called phagocytes (cell "eaters"). Then we'll examine the lymphocytes, also known as T-cells and B-cells. Next comes a peek at the complement system, and finally some words on interferon and interleukin.

Immunity from What?

What threatens your immunity? What is it your immune system protects you from? Antigens. Antigens are viruses, bacteria, cancer cells, fungi, protozoa (microscopic animals), particles, and anything else that challenges your immune system.

Antigens are the reason the immune system exists. If there were no antigens to worry about there would be no need for an immune system.

Not every danger will excite the immune system into action. Some cancers for example, may disguise themselves in such a way that they remain in the body, undetected by the immune system, until it's too late. And of course, antigens don't take being attacked lying down. They have their own weapons, strategies and tricks. Some antigens try to fool the immune system by changing their surface configuration, so they won't be recognized. Others battle the immune system, hoping to overwhelm it. As the microscopic battle rages, millions of our immune soldiers die. The AIDS virus seems particularly adept at crippling the immune system's ability to mount a defense.

How Is the Battle Fought?

So antigens are the enemy, they challenge our immunity, and the immune system fights back. How?

One method of attack is for certain immune cells to "eat" antigens. Another is to cut a hole in the surface of the bacteria's cell. This destroys the bacteria by allowing water, sodium and other substances to leak in and out of the cell, upsetting its homeostasis ("steady state"). Poison can be used to kill the antigen. Or a cover can be slapped over that part of the antigen which does the damage (toxic site).

Some of the immune cells are born knowing how to locate and destroy antigens. Other parts of the immune system must wait until they receive specific instructions, telling them what the antigen looks like.

The brunt of battle falls on the white blood cells, which we call leucocytes. ("Leuco" refers to the color white and "cytes" to the cells.)

Using a video screen hooked up to a microscope, I often show my patients what a drop of their blood looks like. There are lots of circular red blood cells: 5,200,000 per cubic millimeter in normal men, give or take 300,000. (For women the figure is 4,700,000, plus or minus 300,000.) Far less numerous are the white blood cells: only about 7,000 in a cubic millimeter of normal adult blood. There are different kinds of white blood cells, each with its own name, size, shape and function:

> Neutrophils (leucocytes/phagocytes)
> Monocyte/Macrophages (leucocytes/phagocytes)
> Eosinophils (leucocytes/phagocytes)
> Basophils (leucocytes)
> Lymphocytes (leucocytes)
>> T-cells (lymphocytes)
>>> Natural Killer Cells (NKs)
>>> Helper Cells (T4s)
>>> Suppressor Cells (T8s)
>> B-cells (lymphocytes)

White blood cells aren't the only immune soldiers. The complement system, immunoglobulins, interferon and interleukin, which I'll discuss later, are also important parts of your defense network.

ᴠ Cell Eaters

Imagine tiny eating machines slowly moving through your bloodstream, They send out a limblike projection (pseudopod) which acts like a "foot" to pull themselves forward, then push out another "foot" to pull themselves forward, and so on, as they crawl through body tissue in search of antigens. These specialized white blood cells are called phagocytes.

A phagocyte is a cell eater, a cell that literally eats other cells. Phagocytes engulf antigens and kill them with deadly poisons.

Neutrophils and monocyte/macrophages are both phagocytes. Of the approximately 7,000 white blood cells in a cubic millimeter of normal adult blood, about 62 percent are neutrophils, and 5.3 percent are monocytes. Neutrophils are mature phagocytes, ready to eat bacteria, viruses and other antigens. The immature monocytes, on the other hand, are not very effective: not yet.

♣ From Monocytes to Macrophage

The neutrophils and monocyte/macrophages don't remain in the blood stream for long. Soon, they squeeze through tiny pores in the blood vessels, holes smaller than they are. How do they fit? Through a process called diapedesis, which means pushing small parts of themselves through the pore at a time, much the same way you'd work a half-filled water balloon through a hole in a fence.

When they arrive in the tissue, the monocytes begin to grow, swelling to four or five times their original size. As they grow they become more and more powerful, developing extra energy sources and poison packets. Pretty soon, they're giant-sized. To match their new stature comes a new name: macrophage, which means "giant eater."

And giant eaters they are. Neutrophils can only swallow and destroy 5 to 20 antigens before they die of "indigestion." The giant eaters, however, can gobble up as many as 100 antigens. And they eat and kill bigger antigens than the smaller neutrophils do. In fact, one of the macrophages' jobs is to help clear the battlefield by eating up dead neutrophils.

There are more differences between the two kinds of cell eaters. While the neutrophils are constantly on patrol, most of the macrophages stand guard at strategic points in the body. There they remain, giant sentries, for months or even years, our first line of defense against antigens.

Foot Soldiers and Shock Troops

Neutrophils are like foot soldiers. They're lightly armed, and there are plenty of them. When they receive a call to battle, they rush into the fray, often dying by the millions in defense of our health. The bigger, tougher giant eaters are like highly-trained, elite shock troops. There aren't as many of them, but they pack quite a punch. The macrophages can also manufacture a protein called tumor necrosis factor (TNF) that works well against cancer cells.

Another difference between the two types of cell eaters is that neutrophils eat and eat until they die of "antigenic indigestion." You see, they can't excrete what they eat to make room for more. But the giant macrophages eat'em, kill'em, spit'em out and go back for more.

How do the phagocytes know what to attack and what to eat? There are a couple of tests the cell eaters apply. For example, our body cells tend to be smooth. Rough objects are therefore more likely to be attacked than smooth ones. Also, most of the substances that belong to our bodies have an electronegative charge; so do the phagocytes, and negative charges repel each other. Antigens and dead tissue, however, have electropositive charges, which attract the cells eaters. These are just two of the detection methods used by the immune system.

T-Cells and B-Cells

Cell eaters are born knowing what to do, so they can rush right into battle. Other white blood cells, called lymphocytes, hold back, studying the antigen, preparing themselves to join the battle. Why the two approaches? Well, there are numerous antigens, and the antigens are constantly evolving new molecular structures and new ways to attack. It is impossible for the immune system to know which antigens will attack over a lifetime or what new guises they might adopt. So we have two types of immune soldiers: the generalists and the specialists.

Phagocytes are generalists; they'll attack and try to gobble up all the antigens they can. But what if an antigen evolves methods of evading or defeating the phagocytes? That's where the lymphocytes come in. They're specialists, and they are given very specific instructions before they're sent out after antigens.

Special training is a good idea, but it takes time. What's to prevent antigens from wreaking havoc before the lymphocytes are ready? That's where phagocytes come into play. Their job is to defeat the germs or hold them off until the lymphocytes are ready to attack.

What are Lymphocytes?

Lymphocytes are special kinds of white blood cells associated with the lymph tissue of the body. ("Lymph" refers to lymph tissue, "cyte" to cells.) Lymphoid tissue is a specialized complex of tissue in the body.

There are two main categories of lymphocytes: T-lymphocytes and B-lymphocytes. T-lymphocytes are called T-cells because they receive their programming from the thymus gland. Like the phagocytes, T-cells engage the enemy in hand-to-hand combat. B-lymphocytes, called B-cells, are more like artillery. From their positions in the lymph tissue, B-cells set in motion the machinery that manufactures "guided missiles" (antibodies), which home in on and destroy antigens.

The lymphoid tissues of your body, where the T and B-cells "live," include the bone marrow, spleen, gastrointestinal tract, pulmonary tract, tonsils, the many lymph nodes all over the body, and the thymus gland.

(Tap the middle part of your breast bone with your finger. The thymus is located right under your finger.)

Picture a lymph gland in your mind; imagine that it is a fort, full of T-cells and B-cells awaiting instructions. When they get their battle orders, they eagerly study them, scrutinizing and memorizing the features of their enemy: the antigens.

Then an amazing thing happens. Certain T and B-cells swing into action, and the lymphocytic "assembly lines" spew out weapon after weapon. Meanwhile, other lymphocytes are acting like computers, receiving and storing information about these antigens. If they ever come back, your immune system will be ready for them.

What are these marvelous weapons? Sensitized T-cells and B-cell antibodies. Let's begin with a look at the T-cells, then examine the B-cells.

T-Cells in Action

When T-cell colonies in the lymph tissue are exposed to an antigen, some of the T-cells become sensitized. These sensitized cells are sent out to find the antigens. When the antigens are found, the sensitized T-cells surround them and hold on, swelling in size and trying to kill the invaders with poisons they release. Along with the poison, the T-cells send out other chemicals that cause nearby T-cells to become sensitized to the antigen and join the battle. In addition, the chemicals attract up to 1,000 macrophages and increase the phagocytic activity of the giant cell eaters. It was recently reported that certain T-cells shoot out proteins, called perforans, that punch holes in antigens. A T-cell may attach itself to several antigens at a time, swinging its "guns" onto one enemy at a time, attacking each in turn.

Killer, Helper and Suppressor Cells

There are different kind of T-cells: the fighting cells I've just described, the memory cells which store away information about the antigen, plus the very important helper T-cells and suppressor T-cells.

Natural killer cells are powerful, but they need a little prodding. That's where the helper T-cell, also called T4 cells, come in. Their job is to prod fighting T-cells, and B-cells, to battle. Of course, your body wants to make sure there's a way to turn the fighters off when the battle is over. That's where the suppressor (T8) cells come in.

The T8s tell the immune soldiers to lay down their weapons and calm down when the battle is over and won. Without T8 cells, the killer cells might go on fighting when the antigens have been destroyed, and turn against you, attacking your own body.

When Cells Rebel

Sometimes the delicate systems of checks and balances in the body fails, and our fighting cells do turn against us. When this happens, we call the problem an autoimmune disease. One of these diseases, called systemic lupus erythematosus, is an often-fatal illness that afflicts mostly young women. There's also idiopathic ulcerative colitis, which may cause, among other problems, bloody diarrhea. Polyarteritis, a severe disease of the arteries I used to see a lot of, is an autoimmune disease, as is scleroderma, which produces a thickening of the skin, esophagus, lungs, intestinal tract and other body tissues. One of the most horrifying moments I ever experienced as a young doctor was when I touched a patient's arm and his skin came off in my hand. He was suffering from an auto-immune disease called dermatomyositis.

Crushing an Autoimmune Rebellion . . .

This is not easy task. We can, however, often read the signs of a potential problem in the blood. Although the helper cells and suppressor cells look alike, we can measure the amounts of each in a blood sample. I routinely examine these cells in those patients I suspect of having an immune-system malfunction.

Because the T8 (suppressor) cells are designed to keep an eye on the rabble-rousing T4 (helper) cells, the ratio between the two is an important indicator of one's immune-system health.

As I point out in Chapter 11, the T4/T8 ratio should range from about 1.6 to 1.8 (1.6 to 1.8 helper cells for every one suppressor cell). A T4/T8 ratio less than one is a strong indication of an immune abnormality: not enough helper cells to spur the fighting cells into action.

B-Cell Guided Missiles

While the T-cells in the lymph tissue are becoming sensitized to an antigen, certain B-cells begin to grow, change appearance and divide into generations of daughter cells called plasma cells. Plasma cells are like factories that manufacture antibodies. It takes only a few days for a single B-cell to grow into hundreds of plasma cells, each producing thousands and thousands of antibodies that "know" exactly which antigen they're after. Imagine Zeus, the Greek king of gods, standing on Mount Olympus, hurling lightning bolts down to Earth, one after the other. Now picture hordes of plasma cells, throwing antibody after antibody at the invading antigens.

What are these antibodies? They're called immuno-globulins, Ig for short. There are five categories of immunoglobulins: IgA, IgD, IgE, IgG and IgM. Shaped like a tiny "Y," immunoglobulins have a constant portion (the bottom) and a variable portion (the top). It's the variable portion that distinguishes one type of antibody from another.

Roughly 75 percent of the total immunoglobulins in a normal person are IgG. Along with IgMs, IgGs go after bacteria and viruses. IgE, of which there are few, are involved in allergic responses, while IgAs are assigned the task of protecting the mucosa (the lining of the respiratory, gastrointestinal and urogenital tracts). When I want to know if a disease—hepatitis, for example—is recent or old, I look at the IgG and IgM counts. Elevated IgM indicates that the disorder is recent, while increased IgG points to an older problem.

Antibodies have several ways of dealing with antigens. Some strong antibodies can tackle the invader head on, ripping open the cell membrane and killing the antigen. Or the immunoglobulins can neutralize the enemy by covering up its toxic site. Another method is for multiple antibodies to bind themselves to antigens, clumping them together in a big bunch and rendering them harmless. (This is called agglutination.) There are other methods of attack, but antibodies are most effective when they work with other parts of your immune system, such as the complement system.

Immune Protection Complements of the Complement System

Complements are plasma proteins that circulate in the blood. Many complements, such as C1, C2, C3 and so on, make up the complement system. When not engaged in battle, they drift in an inactive state. When activated, the tough little complements line up and go for the kill.

Individually, the various complements can't harm antigens. It takes the right combination, assembled at the right time, in the right place, to act. And assemble they do, at just the proper time and place.

Imagine the complements zeroing in on bacteria. Picture the first little complement attaching itself to the bacteria. The next complement attaches to the first, then another and another. When they're all in place, the bacteria ruptures and dies, its cell wall eaten away by enzymes secreted by the complements.

Complements can also neutralize antigens by attacking their molecular structure; by changing the surfaces of antigens and making them stick together; and by prompting inflammation that will, among other things, block off the antigens so that they can't spread to other parts of the body. The complements can also send out a chemical call for help that brings more neutrophils and macrophages to the scene. At the same time, the complements change the surface features of the antigen in such a way as to make them more "appetizing" to the cell-eaters.

Biochemical Cooperation

The complements aren't the only immune soldiers that work together. T-cells, as you remember, secrete chemicals that increase the cell-eating activity of the giant macrophages. Antibodies assist macrophages by locking onto antigens and identifying them as enemies to be devoured. And macrophages help the lymphocytes (T and B-cells) by acting as "scouts."

Macrophages are stationed right by the lymphocyte colonies in various lymph tissues. It's felt that the macrophages face the antigen first. The macrophages devour the antigen, then excrete a piece of it, which they "present" to the T and B-cells to study. The piece of dead antigen acts like battle orders for the lymphocytes, exciting some of them to action.

The cells of your immune system constantly interact with other cells by releasing substances that "give orders" to other cells. Earlier I mentioned that immune soldiers engaging antigens can send out a chemical "call for help," and that T-cells release chemicals that increase the phagocytic activity of the macrophage, and sensitize other T-cells to the same antigen.

Interferon

Lymphocytes (T and B-cells) also make substances called lymphokines. Interferon is one of the lymphokines. When a cell is attacked by a virus, for example, the cell releases interferon. Interferon interacts with other, uninfected cells, stimulating them to make an antiviral protein that protects the second cell from the virus. Interferon can travel through the blood, casting its protective net over different parts of the body. Interferon prompted by one type of virus can protect cells against other viruses, as well as the original one. What's more, interferons also help regulate other immune cells, for example, by increasing the production of fighting T-cells.

One type of interferon has been tested and used on a number of patients with CMV cytomegalic virus infections and hepatitis, and with AIDS patients who have Kaposi's sarcoma.

Interleukin: From Cell Eater to T-Cell to B-Cell

Another example of immune-system cooperation is interleukin. Macrophages produce a substance called interleukin-I (IL.I), which leads to an increase in T-cells. The T-cells then manufacture interleukin-II (IL-2), which helps get the B-cells producing antibodies.

Interleukin-II has recently been hailed as an amazing breakthrough in the war against cancer. It seems that the immune systems of some cancer patients don't fully mobilize to fight the cancer. For what ever reason, the antigen (cancer) doesn't elicit a full immune response; the immune system doesn't seem to pay proper attention to the problem. New studies have described how scientists took blood from these cancer patients, separated out the lymphocytes and mixed them with interleukin- II. The lymphocyte/interleukin complexes were injected back into the bloodstream, and the rejuvenated lymphocytes were better able to attack the cancer.

An Old Idea—and a New one

Back in my days as a resident in internal medicine at the Los Angeles County Hospital, we didn't have many of the drugs and surgeries that are now used. This was in the late 1950s, before the antibiotic explosion. Penicillin had been introduced in 1945, and other antibiotics were introduced in the fifties, but most of the doctors practicing then had been trained before antibiotics were available.

I remember the older doctors telling me about what they did for some of their patients. They gave these people, who had cancer and other diseases, injections containing extracts of dead bacteria. The idea was that if the patients' immune systems weren't responding to the actual antigen, they would give them another antigen (dead bacteria). The patients, it was hoped, would respond with a fever and full mobilization of the immune system. Thirty years ago these doctors were using our most modern and exciting theories on the immune system. Today we're coming around full circle, utilizing the body's own defenses to fight off invaders.

Lights, More Lights, and Lots of Action

There's more to your immune system than phagocytes, lymphocytes, complements, interferon and interleukin. Imagine you're looking at a life-size picture of the human body. Pretend there are tiny lights flashing on and off all over the body. There are red lights representing the neutrophils, green for the macrophages, yellow for the fighting T-cells and blue for the B-cells. Gray lights mark the complement system that drifts through the blood, and orange lights identify the giant sentry macrophages found all over the body.

But there's more. Add purple lights for the memory cells which remember the features of the antigen, and brown, which represents interferon. Silver lights mark the interleukins, with gold, pink, peach and other colors for immune components such as the prostaglandins, the leukotrines, basophils, eosinophils, histamines, kinins and the other parts of your immune system.

Visualize the whole body covered with lights of every color packed tightly into every corner and crevice, a brilliant display of the immense power your immune system commands. All that healing power is dedicated to health, *your* health.

This brief discussion only begins to explore the immune system. There is now an information explosion concerning the immune system. It's like the universe Einstein described: there's no end to the new information pouring forth. I hope you've learned a little and picked up a bit of the excitement I feel when I think about the miraculous and powerful defense system that nature has created for us. Let's do everything we can to help it to take care of us.

Chapter 10

Immune Alert

*I*n Chapter One I described some of the possible signs and symptoms of immune-system malfunction. Let's take a closer look at a few of the more common immune-system diseases. The signs and symptoms listed aren't necessarily the only signals of the disease, and all of them may not occur in every instance. The point is to give you an idea of what the signs of impending immune difficulty may be.

AIDS: life-threatening, infectious disease spread by sexual contact, and other exchanges of body fluids, such as blood transfusions and intravenous-needle use. Caused by the HIV-I virus, AIDS selectively causes immune suppression by destruction of T4 cells. Presently, it is not known what the incubation time for AIDS's: It may be five years or more. We've only been tracking AIDS for five years or so, so we can't say with absolute confidence that it is or is not easily spread. Presently, AIDS is considered fatal.

Signs and Symptoms: fever; cough; shortness of breath; sweats; enlarged lymph nodes in the neck, groin and other parts of the body; weight loss; often diarrhea; skin rashes; body wasting; muscle loss; may progress on to pneumonia, usually caused by opportunistic infections. Opportunistic infections are often caused by antigens that would ordinarily present little or no problem to our immune system. But with the immune system crippled by AIDS, these organisms cause a great deal of damage. Fifty percent of AIDS victims will have the opportunistic infection pneumocystis carinii pneumonia; about 25 percent or so will have Kaposi's sarcoma (first sign of Kaposi's may be pigmented spots on the skin). A small number will have both pneumocystis carinii and Kaposi's. When you have AIDS, a simple infection such as herpes simplex or thrush mouth *(Candida albicans)* can be life-threatening.

ANKYLOSING SPONDYLITIS: a progressive, inflammatory arthritis characterized by fusion of various joints, especially of the spine, that leads to years of suffering. Norman Cousins described his experience with ankylosing spondylitis in his bestselling book, *Anatomy of an Illness.*

Signs and Symptoms: fatigue; malaise; weight loss; low back pains; sacroiliac pains; sometimes pain down the back of the legs; stiffness of the back, especially in the morning; stiffness and pain spreading up to involve the rest of the back; hips and shoulders ache and feel stiff; in advanced stages there is forward flexion of the spine, forcing the person to walk with his head facing the ground (almost like an exaggerated Groucho Marx walk).

BACTEREMIA: a condition in which bacteria invade the circulating blood. The bacteria can come from a small abcess on the skin, dental drilling or manipulations, infections in the urinary tract or female organs, lung infections, intravenous drug use, indwelling intravenous catheters, urinary catheters, surgical procedures, and almost any other way bacteria can get into your blood.

Signs and Symptoms: fever; fatigue; rapid heart rate; rapid breathing; cool, pale extremities; can lead to confusion or disorientation; shortness of breath.

CANCER: the ultimate failure of the immune system. Whether cancer is fatal or not depends on what type of cancer it is, how soon it is detected and other factors.

Signs and Symptoms: depend on where the cancer is. The first signs and symptoms of a cancer may be fatigue, weakness, lethargy, depression, irritability, vague behavioral changes, loss of appetite, a persistent cough and other general problems. Lung cancer may cause no symptoms for a long time. If the bronchial tubes, rather than the lungs themselves, are involved, an irritating type of cough may be experienced. Stomach cancer may produce no symptoms, or there may be abdominal pains mimicking the pain of gastritis or an ulcer. There may be diarrhea, constipation, vague or severe abdominal pain. Blood may appear in the stool, or the stool may appear black in color (depending on where the bleeding is). Colo-rectal cancer may produce no symptoms until the advanced stages. There may be rectal bleeding (pay attention to any blood in the stool). There may also be a change in bowel habits. The stool may become like "squeezed toothpaste." There may be vague abdominal pains, and, at times, pain upon bending forward.

Ovarian cancer can produce a feeling of "fullness" in the abdomen, and clothes seem a little tighter. Vague to severe pains in the lower abdomen and pelvic area may also occur.

Breast cancer may or may not produce pain. Symptoms of the cancer may be severe or may not appear until later on. There may be tenderness in the breasts, hardening or thickening of the breast or a sore on the breast. A lump may be discovered, and there may be swelling under the arms. The nipple may be ulcerated or inverted (turned in). There may be a discharge from the nipple, which can contain a bloody or a non-bloody fluid.

Pancreatic cancer may cause severe symptoms or no symptoms, although there is generally a loss of appetite and loss of weight as the disease progresses. The cancer may be characterized by severe abdominal pain, often in the center but spreading out to both sides of abdomen. In many cases the pain goes through to the back. In fact, back pain may predominate, causing the person to be treated for a back problem. If the head of the pancreas is involved, the bile ducts can be obstructed, and there is usually a painless jaundice (the skin and the whites of the eyes become yellow, the urine becomes dark and the stool becomes light in color). The liver or gallbladder may enlarge, and pain may be experienced under the lower right ribs or the right upper side of abdomen.

Uterine cancer may be indicated by vaginal bleeding from a woman who hasn't had a period for a long time, or periods may become longer and irregular. There may or may not be pain.

Prostate cancer grows very slowly, so signs and symptoms occur gradually. There may be difficulty in urinating, frequent urination, or some trouble in starting or stopping urination. Later on there may be blood in the urine, pus or obstructions to urination. If the cancer spreads to the bones of the pelvis and lower back, there may be severe pains in those regions. In fact, many low-back problems in men over 65 are due to cancer of the prostate.

CHYLAMYDIAL DISEASES: a common, sexually transmitted infection, which is occurring in epidemic proportions. It can cause sterility in women and problems such as inflammation of the urinary tract and prostatic inflammation in men.

Signs and Symptoms: may be nonexistent, but generally it causes infections of the lining of the uterus, the uterine tubes and ovaries; vaginal discharge; abnormal pap smears; pelvic pain; genital infections; enlarged glands in the groin areas; inflammation of the rectum; fever. The liver and a part of the testicle (epididymis) can be involved. Chylamydial diseases are one of the major causes of sterility in women.

COCCIDIOIDOMYCOSIS: a disease caused by fungus infection, common in the Southwest U.S., which can involve the lungs, skin, lymph nodes, spleen, brain, bones, kidneys or liver. Most cases begin as a flu-like syndrome and may not progress any further.

Signs and Symptoms: depend upon where in the body the fungus is doing the most damage. Generally there is a chronic, low-grade fever; loss of weight; generalized loss of strength; loss of appetite; shortness of breath; cough, which can produce yellow or green sputum; can be aches in joints. If the fungus gets into the brain, there can be destruction of tissue, with confusion and coma. If in the bones, there can be bone pain.

COMMON COLD: a virus that attacks the upper respiratory tract, especially the nose and throat.

Signs and Symptoms: occur one to three days after exposure if the immune system fails to resist the cold. Generally an ache in the throat; runny nose; sneezing; a feeling of malaise. Adults may or may not have fever, children generally do. Often hoarseness of voice; cough due to inflammation of trachea; some tightness of the chest. There may be a burning sensation in the mouth and throat, and there may be discharge (secretions) from throat or nose. A cold generally lasts a week, although it may go into a second week. If it continues longer, suspect a bacterial invasion.

EPSTEIN-BARR VIRUS (EBV): causes infectious mononucleosis. It's been shown in Africa to cause a form of cancer, and it may be a sign of impending immune-system failure. Some studies indicate it's present in many cases of AIDS.

Signs and Symptoms: may be nonexistent or nonspecific such as weakness, fatigue, malaise. Also see mononucleosis.

FUNGAL DISEASES (such as yeast, candidiasis): fungi invade the body.

Signs and Symptoms: possibly fever; malaise; lack of energy; anemia; depression; loss of appetite; cough; vaginal discharge; urinary tract infections; irritability.

FEVER OF UNDETERMINED ORIGIN (FUO): generally a fever that lasts for three weeks without the cause being discovered. FUOs generally have signs and symptoms of the underlying disease, which in the very beginning may be very vague.

Signs and Symptoms: malaise; fatigue; joint and muscle aches; other symptoms, depending on the cause of the fever.

GASTRITIS, ACUTE EROSIVE: superficial inflammation of the lining of the stomach, most commonly caused by aspirin, alcohol, cortisone medications, nonsteroidal, antiinflammatory drugs (often used for arthritis pain). Also caused by toxins (poisons) put out by staphylococcus. Anything that causes stress, such as severe anxiety, severe burns, and multiple-type injuries to other parts of the body, can also prompt gastritis.

Signs and Symptoms: usually loss of appetite; nausea; vomiting; upper abdominal pain; pain after eating. There may also be bleeding; vomiting of blood; black bowel movements.

HERPES SIMPLEX (cold sores, fever blisters):   Type 1 is usually found on the lips and skin. Type 2 is easily transmitted by sexual contact and usually occurs on the genital organs.

Signs and Symptoms: generally begins with the area to be involved looking OK, but there may be tingling, discomfort or a slight ache. Severe pain often occurs. Then a blister or blisters can form. Blisters generally last about a week, break, then crust over. By the third week all signs are completely gone. Herpes can be associated with fever or malaise.

HERPES ZOSTER (shingles):   can occur at any age, most commonly after 50; is not easily communicable.

Signs and Symptoms: fever; weakness; malaise; chills; loss of appetite; nausea. Severe, unremitting pain, resistant to almost all treatment, may occur, following a nerve route. About the fifth day blisters occur following the same nerve route as the pain did, most commonly on the trunk.

HYPOTHYROIDISM: a deficiency of thyroid hormone, most commonly due to Hashimoto's inflammation of the thyroid.

Signs and Symptoms: strike slowly. There is an insidious onset of weakness; fatigue; loss of energy; loss of drive; forgetfulness; personality changes. Skin becomes dry, coarse, scaly, thick; eyelids droop; face assumes a dull expression; puffiness and swelling around eyes; feet swell; hands and feet may become numb and tingly. Heavy menstrual periods and low body temperature also occur.

INFECTION WITH CYTOMEGALOVIRUS (CMV): viral infection which over 60 percent of adults may have at one time or another. May be without consequence or can be serious. Can lead to hepatitis, cause abortion, stillbirth, liver damage. Can be found in immune-compromised people; may be a pre-AIDS condition.

Signs and Symptoms: can be symptomless or can be characterized by fever; tiredness; malaise; weakness; gland enlargement in the neck and elsewhere, with or without pain.

INFLUENZA (flu, grippe):   viral invasion, usually of

the lining of the respiratory tract. May spread to other parts of the body, such as the blood or gastrointestinal tract.

Signs and Symptoms: fever of sudden onset, 102-103 degrees; general chills; aches all over, especially in back and legs; headache; weakness; sensitivity to light; often aching behind eyes; watery discharge from eyes; whites of eyes may be reddened; sore throat; dry cough, although later may cough up mucous; the skin is flushed; often runny nose.

LEGIONNAIRES' DISEASE: caused by bacteria *Legionella Pneumophila.* Many victims died during the initial outbreak of the disease, but it can be treated today.

Signs and Symptoms: generally begins with high fever, which increases over a couple of days. May be severe weakness; disorientation; confusion; loss of appetite; often prostration; dry cough (not bad at first). Later on, cough can be watery or even have some blood in it. The heart rate is slow with this high fever, and there are chills of the shaking type. There can be pain of the chest on breathing. Watery diarrhea is common. Other signs and symptoms include headache; possible shortness of breath; aches in the muscles and joints; nausea; vomiting; sore throat; may be (but not commonly) a runny nose.

LUPUS ERYTHEMATOSUS, SYSTEMIC: an inflammatory disease of connective tissue, occurring mostly in young women. Believed to be an autoimmune disease. May progress over a long period of time and may ultimately lead to death in some cases.

Signs and Symptoms: fever and malaise, which can progress insidiously over a period of years; joint pains; joint swelling may occur; allergic-like skin eruptions or various skin rashes; a "butterfly" rash on the face; loss of hair; redness of the palms; spontaneous bruises may occur; pleurisy; chest pains; pericarditis (inflammation of the sac surrounding the heart); endocarditis (inflammation of the inner lining of the heart); swelling of the lymph glands; symptoms of small strokes (transient weakness or paralysis of extremities, momentarily forgetfulness, etc.); patients may have depression, epileptic convulsions, dementia, confusion and many other symptoms.

MULTIPLE SCLEROSIS (MS): a progressive disease of the central nervous system, characterized by loss of the covering of nervous tissue (demyelination) of the brain and spinal cord. MS may lead to a weakened condition, which, in turn, leads to death.

Signs and Symptoms: weakness; fatigue; dizziness; weakness of hands or legs; transitory weakness or stiffness of a limb or extremity. Difficulty in walking may occur. May be pain in an extremity, also numbness and tingling. May be pain in one eye, blurring or dimness of vision. Problems with bladder control may occur. Victim may be easily upset emotionally. May be a tendency toward slow, hesitant speech. Disease is characterized by periods of advancing symptoms, then remission.

MONONUCLEOSIS: formerly called the kissing disease. Caused by the EB virus.

Signs and Symptoms: may last a week to a month, or may linger for several months. Symptoms include fatigue; weakness; headaches; irritability; chills, then a fever, which may be high. Sore throat often predominates at this point. Glands enlarge, especially glands in the neck. Liver tests are generally abnormal, and liver may be enlarged in some people. Spleen (under the left front ribs) is enlarged in about half those with mononucleosis. Often there is a red rash that passes quickly, and there may be little red spots inside the mouth on the hard and soft palate. Rarely, there may be a cough or chest pain. The disease can involve the brain, and not commonly lead to encephalitis and other brain inflammations.

PEPTIC ULCER: most commonly found in the first part of the intestine (called the duodenum) and also in the stomach and esophagus. Usually occurs in adults, although it can strike children as well.

Signs and Symptoms: pain, which may begin as a hunger pang or an "empty feeling." This may progress to a soreness, then an aching and gnawing feeling, on to a burning sensation and possibly severe pain. Often there is bleeding from the ulcer, causing black colored stool, or there may be vomiting of blood. Pain is usually located in the upper-middle portion of the abdomen, but can occur in other places. Eating usually brings pain relief. Patients often wake up in the middle of the night with abdominal pain.

RHEUMATIC FEVER: streptococcal infection of the throat, which then attacks joints and the heart. Usually occurs in children.

Signs and Symptoms: skin rash; pains in joints; swelling of joints; malaise; fatigue; lethargy. Can cause heart murmurs. May be vague abdominal pain. People used to call the joint pains "growing pains."

RHEUMATOID ARTHRITIS: chronic inflammation of joints.

Signs and Symptoms: fatigue; malaise; early morning stiffness of joints and muscles. Swelling of joints occurs, usually starting in the small joints such as hands, feet, ankles, wrists, elbows, although it can occur in any joint. Usually both sides of the body are affected simultaneously (for example, both wrists or both elbows). Deformities of joints can occur, and contractures of joints are also seen. Fever may be present. Lungs may also be affected.

ROCKY MOUNTAIN SPOTTED FEVER: caused by the bite of a tick carrying the germ *Rickettsia*. It's called Rocky Mountain Spotted Fever, but it has been found in almost every state.

Signs and Symptoms: occur suddenly. Headaches; fever; chills; pains in muscles; pains in joints; cough that usually produces no sputum. A rash, first appearing on the extremities, then the rest of the body including the neck and face. Victim can develop severe lethargy; weakness; difficulty in sleeping; pneumonia; can become delirious, may even fall into coma.

SARCOIDOSIS: we don't know what causes it; possibly a virus.

Signs and Symptoms: may be fever; pains in joints; generalized body aches; cough; weight loss. Can have shortness of breath, lumps on the skin; enlarged liver; inflammation of a portion of the eye, which can lead to glaucoma and loss of vision. May get into heart and cause chest pain. Usually gets into lungs, causing shortness of breath. Many times I have made the diagnosis of sarcoidosis from the characteristic appearance of the X-ray, which shows enlarged lymph glands in the chest.

SCLERODERMA (progressive systemic sclerosis):   chronic disease with generalized fibrosis (thickening) of the skin, joints and many internal organs.

Signs and Symptoms: joint pains; stomach upsets; heartburn; weight loss; malaise; difficulty in swallowing; shortness of breath. Skin of fingers and face becomes thick. Normal creases on the fingers and face disappear. Fingers become purple and hurt when exposed to cold. Face become thick, like a mask, and blood vessels on face, lips and tongue become prominent. Other symptoms may be esophagitis; (inflammations of the esophagus); pleurisy,; pericarditis (inflammation of the sac surrounding the heart);

heart irregularities; muscle weakness. Death from pneumonia often occurs.

TOXIC SHOCK SYNDROME (TSS): lately associated with the use of vaginal tampons, although 15 percent of cases occur in men. It's an infection of *Staphylococcus aureus*, and can involve the mouth, nose, vagina and trachea. Many fatalities have been associated with TSS.

Signs and Symptoms: sudden fever that can remain high, up to 105 degrees. Also headache; discharge from eyes; sore throat; severe weakness and malaise; watery diarrhea; vomiting; redness of skin almost like acute sunburn; intermittent confusion. Symptoms may progress to shock and, in some cases, death. By the end of a week, some of the skin that was so red, especially skin on the palms of the hands and soles of the feet, may slough off.

TUBERCULOSIS: caused by bacteria called *Mycobacterium tuberculosis*. Can occur in any part of body, but usually strikes the lungs. Symptoms vary with part of body affected.

Signs and Symptoms: first symptoms include coughing up of blood; shortness of breath; fever. Signs and symptoms depend upon where the bacteria settles in the body. Constitutional signs and symptoms include fever; malaise; loss of appetite; weight loss; haggard appearance. Tuberculosis is more prevalent in the lungs. May cause cough; a bloody cough; shortness of breath; chest pain; fever; malaise; weight loss. If it's in kidneys, urine may be bloody or filled with pus. In the brain, it can cause changes in behavior, headaches, coma, stupor, drowsiness, death. If it gets into the intestinal tract, can cause abdominal pain and diarrhea. In the adrenals, it can cause adrenal insufficiency (weakness, fatigue and other symptoms). This is called Addison's disease. (President Kennedy suffered from Addison's disease.) If it gets in liver, may cause jaundice. In the joints, it can cause pain and symptoms of arthritis. If in the spine, it may cause backache; collapse of vertebrae. It can invade glands all over the body, especially in the neck.

VIRAL PNEUMONIA: viral infection that involves the lungs and respiratory passages. In schools and the military, viral pneumonia is responsible for 75 percent of all lung infections. CMV and herpes are two of the many viruses that can cause viral pneumonia.

Signs and Symptoms: usually headache; loss of appetite; fever; aches in muscles. Patient feels weak and tired. There is a cough, usually with yellow sputum; rarely bloody.

The diseases I have listed aren't meant to be a representative cross section. They are simply a few of the immune-system problems I've treated over the past 30-plus years. Any of the signs and symptoms I've described could signal impending immune-system failure.

For all its prowess, the immune system is very fragile. There are so many ways to harm it. And the signs and symptoms of immune-system failure may not become evident until the disease is firmly entrenched in your body. An innocent cough that lasts too long may be nothing. But what if it's signaling tuberculosis or cancer? And that fever—is it nothing, or the first sign of AIDS? That's why I feel it's so important to get persistent signs and symptoms checked out by a physician, even if they seem trivial. Better still, adopt the Immune for Life program and prevent the signs and symptoms from occurring.

Chapter 11

More About Vitamins, Minerals and Your Immune System

*A*ll vitamins, minerals, amino acids and other nutrients are vitally important to your immune system. After all, the glands, cells and proteins that make up your immune system use the same building blocks as the other parts of your body. Certain nutrients, however, stand out for the special effects they have on the immune system. Let's take a closer look at these nutrients. This discussion is meant to introduce you to the relationship between certain nutrients and the immune system, not to provide a supplementation program.

Vitamin A

Way back in the 1930s, we knew that vitamin A (also called retinol) modulated the body's defense mechanisms against infection. Vitamin A is especially important in helping to keep fit the parts of our body that are the first to come in contact with invading organisms: the skin and the linings of the respiratory tract, digestive tract, urogenital tract and eyes. These areas of the body are our first line of defense against disease, so it's important for us to get enough vitamin A to keep them strong and healthy. Vitamin A also helps the immune soldiers that are located in your tears and sweat.

If you don't take in enough vitamin A to keep these areas of your body strong, disease-causing organisms that ordinarily would be kept out of your body will find their way in. That's why vitamin A has been nicknamed the "anti-infection" vitamin. Studies have shown that taking substantial amounts of vitamin A helps people resist dangerous invaders.

Vitamin A enhances the activity of the natural killer (NK) cells that are such an important part of your immune system. Natural killer cells are T-cells that engage germs in "hand-to-hand" combat. Vitamin A also enhances the effectiveness of your B-cells. As I explained in Chapter 8, B-cells are the parts of the immune system that produce plasma cells. The plasma cells then manufacture antibodies, which are like guided missiles that seek out and destroy germs.

Vitamin A comes in two forms: preformed vitamin A from fish, meat, poultry, dairy products and other foods of animal origin, and beta carotene from vegetables, fruits and other foods of plant origin. When you eat foods that contain beta carotene, your body converts the carotene into vitamin A as it is needed.

B Complex

The B-complex family of vitamins has been studied extensively. It has been shown that animals and humans who are low in B vitamins have much less resistance to infections. Many of my patients who have suffered from recurrent infections have had low blood levels of some of the B complex vitamins.

Vitamin B6 (Pyridoxine)

Vitamin B_6 has the most immune-system bolstering functions of all the B vitamins. Years ago we found that tuberculosis patients treated with the drug INH (isoniazid) developed severe immune-system problems. It turned out that the INH was altering B_6 levels in the patients, which, in turn, upset their immune systems.

B_6 (as well as B_2 and B_3, to a lesser extent) is important for the synthesis of nucleic acids and protein. The immune system, as well as the rest of the body, is absolutely dependent on adequate supplies of nucleic acids and protein. Without them, your immune defenses would quickly falter.

A deficiency of B_6 leads to shrinking of the thymus gland. It's in the thymus gland, as I pointed out, that the sturdy germ-fighting T-cells receive their programming, so healthy thymus is a vital part of your defense system. A lack of B_6 can harm your immune system in others ways, too, such as prompting a decrease in the total number of T-cells in the blood and upsetting the ratio of T-cells to B- cells.

Vitamin B_{12} and Folic Acid

Many years ago a general practitioner sent me a patient who was suffering from recurrent infections, anemia, numbness and tingling of her extremities. Recurrent infections are a sign that the immune system isn't doing its job well. It turned out that the anemia and other symptoms were caused by a lack of vitamin B_{12} and folic acid. (Folic acid is also a member of the B family of vitamins). She got plenty of B_{12} from her diet, but couldn't properly absorb the B_{12} she ate. We managed to adjust her B_{12} levels and then her folic acid. This served to restart her immune system and eliminate the puzzling symptoms and anemia.

Both B_{12} and folic acid are necessary if the immune-system cells made in the bone marrow are to mature into active disease-fighters. A deficiency of vitamin B_{12} and folic acid is associated with a decrease in the number of neutrophils, immune fighters that "eat" and destroy bacteria and other dangerous particles. Lack of B_{12} results in decreased "cell eating" (phagocytosis), and a fall in the absolute number of T and B-cells. Folic-acid deficiency leads to a decrease in T-cells, as well as shrinkage of the thymolymphatico organs, where so much of your immune system is "based."

Vitamin B5 (Pantothenic acid)

My own studies, and the work of others, have shown that vitamin B5 is positively related to the health of the immune system. Persons deficient in B5, for example, suffer from poor wound healing. One of B5's jobs is to facilitate the release of antibodies from the plasma cells. Antibodies, as you remember, are like guided missiles that travel through your body to destroy disease-causing antigens. Lack of adequate B5 decreases thymolymphatico tissue, decreases the number of immunoglobulins in the blood, and upsets the T- to B-cell ratio.

Vitamin B2 (Riboflavin)

One of vitamin B2's jobs is to help keep the mucosal lining of your body in shape to ward off invaders. The mucosal lining is among our first barriers against disease, so it's important to keep it strong. Deficiencies of B2 are associated with several immune system weaknesses, such as deficits in antibody production, decreases in the numbers of T and B-cells in the blood and shrinkage of thymolymphatico tissue.

Vitamin B1 (Thiamine)

A lack of sufficient B1 can lead to immune-system deficiency, such as lessened resistance to infection, reduced numbers of T- and B-cells, decreased spleen-cell response and a small shrinkage of the thymus. But the effects of a B1 deficit on the immune-system are not as pronounced as those seen because of B6, B12 or folic acid shortage.

Although vitamin B1 has only a mild immune-system enhancing effect, it is very important for general health, energy, growth, muscles and nerves. I have used B1 many times to relieve the symptoms of neuritis (a burning and tingling feeling often felt in the extremities or tongue).

Biotin

Biotin is a member of the B-complex family of vitamins. Scientists now are beginning to look at its effects on the immune system. When children with a rare biotin-deficiency disease were studied, the administration of biotin, in large amounts, also corrected their immune-system weakness. Most of us don't have this rare disease, but the study serves as a model for what we can learn about the effects of biotin, as well as other vitamins and minerals, on the immune system.

B's on the Brain

As a group, the B vitamins are especially important for maintaining a positive outlook on life. Deficits of various B vitamins can lead to anxiety, irritability, nervousness, depression and personality changes. A deficiency of vitamin B_3, in fact, leads to pellagra, a disease that used to be common in the southern regions of this country. Pellagra's signs and symptoms include the "4 Ds": diarrhea, dermatitis, dementia and, in many cases, death.

As we learned earlier, there are strong physical and biochemical links between your mind and body. Your thoughts have a profound influence on the health of your immune system and on other parts of your body. Happy, positive thoughts promote a strong immune system and good health. Negative, unhappy thoughts actually depress the immune system and encourage disease.

So the B vitamins, by helping to keep you happy and positive, have a beneficial effect on your immune system. A deficiency of B vitamins, which leads to unhappiness and personality changes, harms your immune system.

Vitamin C

Years ago, when Nobel prize winner Dr. Linus Pauling announced that vitamin C has a beneficial effect on the immune system, I was unimpressed. Like many other medical doctors, I had little faith in vitamins. But as I studied vitamin C and saw the effects it had on patients, I became convinced that vitamin C is necessary for good immune-system functioning. Some years ago, when I met Dr. Pauling, I was pleased to tell him that he had helped me see the power of vitamin C. More importantly, his work increased my awareness of the health-giving properties of vitamins and minerals in general.

There is a genetic disorder called Chediak-Higashi disease, which is highlighted by a marked lowering of resistance to bacterial infections. Patients who have this disease suffer from recurrent tissue abscesses, sinusitis and pneumonia, all of which are difficult to treat, and the disease is often fatal. Their white blood cell count drops, and the killing power of the cells is reduced. This is a dangerous sign, because the white blood cells bear the brunt of defending the body against disease. Vitamin C has corrected the problem in many patients studied, and it therefore serves as a model for the use of nutrients in helping the immune system to function effectively.

Vitamin C also improves the mobility of white blood cells. Using a video camera and screen hooked up to a microscope, I have seen sluggish white blood cells taken from patients with recurrent infections. After giving these people an injection of vitamin C, I put a fresh sample of their blood under the microscope and watched as the previously "lazy" white blood cells moved about energetically.

Vitamin C has been used to speed up recovery from pneumonia, mononucleosis, hepatitis and almost all viral infections. Studies are underway to evaluate vitamin C as an interferon-releasing agent. (A natural substance produced by your lymphocytes, interferon is involved in the battle against virus and cancer.) Vitamin C stimulates T and B-cells, as well as the giant "cell eaters" (macrophages) which gobble up and destroy bacteria, viruses, fungi and other disease-causing antigens. In addition, vitamin C is an antioxidant and scavenger of free radicals. (Oxidation of molecules in your body is analogous to the rusting of a piece of iron. See vitamin E, below, for more information on free radicals.)

Vitamin D

Vitamin D is necessary for a healthy immune system; a deficiency will hamper the "cell eating" (phagocytic) functions of the white blood cells. In large amounts, however, vitamin D can suppress the immune system.

Vitamin D is made in your body by the action of sunlight on the skin. This vitamin is also added to milk, milk products and flour. Most people get enough vitamin D naturally. I don't generally recommend more than the RDA of vitamin D for my patients unless a condition such as osteoporosis makes it necessary.

Check with your physician before taking vitamin D supplements.

Vitamin E

Vitamin E is very important to your immune system, but too much can reduce immune system effectiveness. Along with vitamins A, B_1, B_5, C and the mineral selenium, vitamin E is a free radical scavenger. Free radicals are tiny killers, even smaller than viruses. Like little chain saws, they destroy cell membranes in your body, causing all sorts of damage, including cancer and damage to your immune system.

Free radicals are formed as by-products of our metabolism. We also get free radicals from the polluted air we breathe. Of course, our bodies make substances to contain free radicals. Along with enzymes called SOD (superoxide dismutase) and glutathione peroxidase, vitamin E and the other nutrients I've mentioned help control the free radicals. The trick is to make sure you have enough free-radical quenchers to keep the free radicals from doing excessive damage.

A deficiency of vitamin E in animals leads to low levels of antibodies, T and B-cells, as well as to decreases in lymphatic organ size and weight. Administering vitamin E to laboratory animals boosts their immune systems' ability to produce antibodies. The "cell eating" activity of the white blood cells is also increased by vitamin E. Some studies have shown that vitamin E may help to counteract the immunosuppressive effects of cortiosteroids (hormones that are associated with depression).

Zinc

Zinc, which has been studied more extensively than any other mineral, has a profound effect on the immune system. As an essential cofactor in more than 100 enzymes, zinc has its "fingers" in a lot of pies. Wounds on animals put on a zinc- deficient diet heal with difficulty, which is an indication of immune-system failure. The animals also suffer from lack of growth, sexual immaturity and loss of hair.

Good supplies of zinc are essential for a healthy immune system. A deficiency of this mineral can lead to shrinkage of the thymus gland, which, in turn, prompts a reduction in the number of T-cells available to grapple with germs. I have found that the ratio of T4 to T8 cells may be skewed as the result of a zinc deficiency. B-cells are adversely affected by a deficiency of zinc, as is the ability of immune-system cells to rush to the scene of a battle and jump into the fight.

Low levels of zinc increase one's susceptibility to infections, and may lead to low levels of blood immunoglobulins. In many cases, administration of zinc restores these immune-system functions to normal levels. I have successfully used a combination of zinc and vitamin C for treating patients with burns or severe wounds. In one case, a 40 year-old woman came to the hospital with severe burns on her legs. The burned skin and muscle were surgically cut away. When the wounds refused to heal, I administered zinc and vitamin C orally, and the stubborn wounds quickly began to heal.

But too much zinc can *depress* the phagocytic activity of neutrophils, so be careful not to overdose on zinc.

Selenium

After zinc, selenium is, I believe, the most important mineral as far as the immune system is concerned. Working with and potentiating the power of vitamin E, selenium is an excellent antioxidant and scavenger of the dangerous free radicals in the body.

As an antioxidant, selenium helps protect cell walls from oxidation. Selenium also helps antagonize mercury and cadmium. These two heavy metals, which enter the body through food, dental fillings, inhalation of paint, and so on, have a deleterious effect on the immune mechanism. Selenium increases cell-eating activity against bacteria, as well as the capacity of macrophages to kill tumors. In laboratory animals, selenium improves antibody response to various antigens and protects against cancer.

Selenium deficiency is associated with a definite drop of the B-cell (antibody) response, delaying its appearance and resulting in lower levels of antibodies.

Iron

A low blood/body level of iron is the most common mineral deficiency in the world. Iron is part of the hemoglobulin molecule that binds oxygen to red blood cells. A lack of iron can result in poor oxygen delivery to the various parts of the body. This can cause all sorts of problems, including immune-system deficits.

In the absence of adequate iron, the thymus and other lymphoid glands may shrink, the number of T and B-cells in the blood can fall, and the ability of cell "eaters" to ingest and destroy bacteria may be impaired. The ability of the body to respond to antigen challenge is thus diminished.

Years ago, doctors gave iron tonics to patients who suffered from multiple infections. The tonics helped, but today we know that iron shouldn't automatically be given to patients with low blood levels of iron.

Bacteria need iron to flourish. So, during infections, the body sequesters iron in the bone marrow and other organs to keep it away from the bacteria. That's pretty smart of the body, hiding the bacteria's food. For this reason, I advise my patients not to take iron when they're suffering from an infection.

If you have symptoms of anemia (such as fatigue), don't self-medicate by taking iron or anything else, for that matter. The anemia may be caused by a serious medical problem that requires attention. In men, the problem may be cancer of the colon, gastritis, esophagitis or peptic-ulcer disease. Taking iron may make you feel better, but it won't do anything for the underlying problem. And because you feel better, you may not seek the treatment you need. Women should also be checked out when suffering from symptoms of anemia. This may sound like a very conservative approach, but through the years I've seen too many people who treated their anemia by taking iron, not knowing until it was too late that the anemia was caused by a serious medical condition that could have been corrected had it been attended to earlier. Too much iron can also be a problem, and it may suppress the immune system.

Copper

There is only a small amount of copper in the body, but it finds its way into many of the body's chemical interactions. Copper is part of the SOD (superoxide dismutase) molecule which scavenges the dangerous free radicals. As part of SOD, copper helps protect against cancer.

You also need copper to properly utilize the iron in

your body. If you don't have enough copper, and cannot make use of the iron you take in, you may find yourself suffering from an iron-deficiency anemia. Anemia, in turn, harms the immune system and other parts of the body. Lack of copper also prompts a weakness of the T-cells and the complement system. The complement system, which I discussed earlier, works with the cell "eaters," T-cells, and other parts of your immune system to destroy bacteria, viruses and other dangerous particles.

Copper and zinc have a "seesaw" effect on each other: too much of one lowers the levels of the other. So don't overdose on either; keep them in balance.

Magnesium

There is plenty of evidence to indicate that the immune system suffers in animals who are deprived of magnesium. A deficit of magnesium causes an unhealthy enlargement of the thymus, which leads to reduced T and B-cell response. Some of the immunoglobulins may also be lowered. An increased incidence of a particular cancer, called malignant lymphoma, has been reported in magnesium-deficient animals.

Like copper, magnesium helps to fight free radicals and cancer as part of the SOD molecule.

Magnesium intake has been reported to be low in the general population, especially among our elderly members.

Manganese

A great deal of research has focused on the relationship between manganese and the immune system in animals. Growth and reproduction are greatly reduced by a manganese deficit. Adequate manganese in the body allows antibody levels to elevate in response to challenges. Manganese is important to humans as well, for it is part of the very important SOD molecule that protects the body against free radicals.

Chapter 12

Understanding Immune-System Tests

The immune-system laboratory tests I listed in Chapter Seven, Nutri-Prevention, give your doctor an idea of how your immune system is functioning. Here's an explanation of what the tests are, what they measure and what the results may mean. Let me caution you once again not to make a diagnosis on the basis of laboratory tests. These tests must be interpreted within the context of your doctor's other findings.

As you read through the tests, you'll be seeing some of these abbreviations:

gm = gram	mcg = microgram
mg = milligrams	mm = millimeters
dl = deciliter	pg = picogram
IU = International Unit	ng = nanogram
cc = cubic centimeter	

White Blood Cell Count

The white blood cell count (WBC) is always included as part of the laboratory work done in a doctor's office, lab or hospital. White blood cells are part of your immune system; they include the T-cells and B-cells that seek out specific antigens, the cell "eaters" and other immune soldiers. A low WBC is often an indication of an unhealthy immune system. After all, you want to have enough immune soldiers to take on disease. A high WBC may be a sign of infection or some other problem causing the body to produce extra white blood cells.

Results: In most labs the WBC ranges from 5,000 to 10,000 per dl for normal people.

Total Lymphocytes

Lymphocytes are the T- and B-cells, special kinds of white blood cells associated with your body's lymph tissue. When the laboratory sends the results of your blood tests to your physician, it will tell him or her what the WBC count is and what percentage of those are lymphocytes. We doctors simply multiple the WBC by the percentage of lymphocytes to determine the number of lymphocytes.

Let's say your WBC is approximately 7,000 per cc of blood, and the percentage of lymphocytes is 30 percent:

        7,000 WBC
    x   .3 .3 = 30% lymphocytes
        2,100 Number of lymphocytes
               per cc of blood

Results: In healthy people, the lymphocyte count should be greater than 2,500. One-third of malnourished patients have counts between 1,500 and 2,500. Less than 1,500 is associated with greater death rates in surgical and other medical patients. Some people who have counts of less than 1,200 have no obvious disease, but they don't feel good. I have seen many chronically ill patients with lymphocyte counts of 1,000 or less. Low lymphocyte counts are associated with immune system problems.

Total T-Cells

T-cells are powerful immune soldiers. They are the natural killer T-cells which tackle the antigens; the helper T-cells, which spur the immune system to battle; and the suppressor T-cells that tell the others when the fight is over. T-cells are effective in fighting viruses, bacteria, fungi, parasites and cancer.

You want to have the proper number of T-cells available at all times. Studies have shown that T-cells are reduced when immune function is diminished, and also in those people suffering from a nutritional deficiency.

Results: Approximately 75 percent of your total lymphocytes should be T-cells, with B-cells accounting for the remaining 25 percent.

T4 to T8 Ratio

This critical ratio looks at the relationship between helper (T4) and suppressor (T8) T-cells. Like everything else in your body, they are delicately balanced, with the helper cells prodding parts of the immune system to action, and the suppressor cells guarding against overreaction. Too few helper cells, and your immune system may fail to respond adequately to an antigen. Too few suppressor cells, and your immune system may turn on you. When this happens, you may contract an autoimmune disease, such as rheumatoid arthritis.

Results: Ordinarily, there are almost two T4 (helper) cells for every one T8 (suppressor) cell. A range of ratios, between 1.6 and 1.8 T4 to one T8, is considered a good balance between the two types of cells.

Lower ratios, 1.5 to 1 down to 1.0 to 1, may be seen with various viral diseases that are knocking the immune system back. Generally, ratios below 1.0 to 1 are seen with a battered immune system.

An elevated T4/T8 ratio may point to an autoimmune disease, inflammatory response, infection, allergy or other disorders.

Immunoglobulins

As I pointed out on page 277, immunoglobulins (Igs) are the antibodies that travel through your body in search of antigens. When B-cells are alerted to the presence of antigens, they produce plasma cells, which, in turn, churn out antibodies specifically programmed to destroy the antigens.

There are five main immunoglobulins: IgA, IgD, IgE, IgG and IgM. I often look at the levels of three immunoglobulins in the blood, IgG, IgA and IgM, which are sufficiently indicative measurements. (An easy way to remember this is to think of GAM.)

Results: For adults,

IgG   600-1600 mg/dl
IgA   76-390 mg/dl
IgM   40-345 mg/dl

Complements

The complement system, as we've seen, is a vital part of your immune system, whether working on its own or teaming up with other immune fighters. The different complements (called C1, C2, C3, C4, etc.) line up in just the right order to attack, boring holes in invading organisms, altering their molecular structure and otherwise making their life difficult. I look at complement C3, the complement that has been studied the most. It takes less than a month of poor eating to bring C3 down to about 60 percent of normal.

Results: Complement C3 is usually between 80 and 155 mg/dl.

Vitamins and Minerals

In addition to the protein and immune function tests, I often look at the levels of these vitamins in the blood: vitamin A, beta carotene, vitamin B_1, vitamin B_2, vitamin B_6, vitamin C and vitamin E. I may also check zinc levels in the blood, and iron is also included in my regular test panel.

As I pointed out earlier, a deficiency of even a single vitamin or mineral can hamper the immune system. Lack of B_1 may cause an increase in infections. A shortage of

B_2 is associated with depressed antibody formation. A deficit of B_6 impairs nucleic acid synthesis and leads to a depression in delayed hypersensitivity reactions. Lowered levels of zinc in the blood are associated with depressed T-cell function (cell-mediated immunity).

Results:	Average Range	Preferred Range
Vitamin A	65-275 IU/100 ml	200-300
Beta carotene	50-250 mcg/dl	250-300
Vitamin B_1	2.0-10.0 mcg/dl	5.0-15.0+
Vitamin B_2	2.6-3.7 mcg/dl	4.0-5.0+
Vitamin B_3	3.0-5.0 mcg/dl	4.0-5.0+
Vitamin B_6	3.8-18.0 ng/ml	5.0-25.0+
Folic acid (Folate)	1.70-15.5 ng/ml	10-20+
Vitamin B_{12}	200-900 pg/dl	500-1000+
Vitamin C (Ascorbic acid)	.20-2.0 mg/dl	1.5-2.5
Vitamin E (tocopherol)	.50-1.50 mg/dl	1.0-2.0
Iron	50-150 mcg/dl	about 100
Zinc	70-130 mcg/dl	about 100

I've included the average range so that you might compare it to my Preferred Range.

Cholesterol

Excess cholesterol is bad for your immune system and dangerous for your "doctor within." As I said earlier, I like to see my patients with a cholesterol of 100 plus their age. Thus, a healthy 45-year-old person should have a cholesterol of about 145. I tell my patients that their cholesterol should certainly be no higher than 150-180 mg/dl.

HDL

HDL (high-density lipoprotein) is the "good" cholesterol I discussed back in Chapter Two. It's felt that HDL acts like a garbage truck, picking up cholesterol from the blood and walls of the arteries and carrying it away. I like to see HDL levels of 45 mg/dl or higher.

LDL

LDL (low-density lipoprotein) is the "bad" cholesterol that seems to function as a delivery truck, bringing cholesterol to the arteries for deposit. I prefer my patients to have LDLs of 100 mg/dl or less.

Coronary Artery Disease Risk Factor

The Coronary Artery Disease Risk Factor (CADRF) is determined by dividing total cholesterol by HDL. For example, if your total cholesterol is 150 and your HDL is 50, your CADRF is 3:

$$CARDF = \frac{150}{50} = 3$$

The higher the CADRF, the greater your chance of suffering a heart attack. For men, a CADRF of:

3.43 = one half the average risk of coronary artery disease.
4.97 = the average risk of coronary artery disease.
9.55 = two times the average risk of coronary artery disease.
23.39 = three times the average risk of coronary artery disease.

For women, a CADRF of:

3.27 = one half the average risk of coronary artery disease.
4.44 = the average risk of coronary artery disease.
7.05 = two times the average risk of coronary artery disease.
11.04 = three times the average risk of coronary artery disease.

But remember: average is awful! You don't want to

have the average risk of suffering from coronary-artery disease. You want your changes to be much better than that.

For men, the CARDF should be 3.5 or less. For women, 3.0 or less is good. The higher the CARDF, the greater your chance of having a heart attack.

Triglycerides

Triglycerides are the fats in your blood. High blood fat is deleterious to your "doctor within" and to your immune system. I tell my patients to keep their triglycerides below 100 mg/dl.

Protein

One of the most important things we doctors can evaluate in the blood is protein. The enzyme systems that keep the body running depend on protein. And the immune system cells, like all cells, can't exist without protein.

"But, Dr. Fox," some patients protest, "didn't you say that the average person gets too much protein?" Yes, I do feel that most of us take in plenty of protein. Still, protein malnutrition is seen in hospitalized patients, in those with colitis, cancer, pancreatitis, chronic illnesses, in alcoholics, persons on fad diets, people taking drugs and others. Protein calorie malnutrition (PCM) is more common than one would think it would be in the Western world. Unfortunately, it's an often overlooked medical-nutritional problem.

Twenty-five to 50 percent of all adults admitted to a hospital for medical or surgical reasons develop signs of PCM within two weeks after admission. I have seen many patients living on nothing but intravenous solutions of five percent glucose in water for a week, ten days, or many weeks.

PCM can occur even where there is plenty of food to eat. There may be excessive food, but it is of limited variety and very low in protein. Years ago a 35-year-old woman was referred to me by another doctor. She complained of weakness and had anemia. Taking her personal and medical history, I learned that this mother of three small children was extremely poor. She and her children ate lots of potatoes—fried, boiled, baked, mashed—and some white rice. Potatoes are good for you, but a diet of mostly potatoes is unhealthy. She and her children were overweight: full, but malnourished. With plenty of calories to eat, but not enough protein, the woman and her children wound up with PCM.

Elderly people who eat only a few different foods, mostly from cans or packages, can also run into trouble. It's wonderful to see how bright and energetic these people become when they are fed correctly. Thus, as part of the Immuno-Nutritional series of blood tests, I look at three proteins in the blood: retinol-binding protein, transferrin and albumin. Both retinol-binding protein and transferrin are sensitive indicators of a person's protein status, because they're rapid-turnover proteins. This means that the body quickly manufactures and destroys the proteins, so a shortage of building blocks (amino acids) will affect these proteins sooner than it will longer-lived proteins. These two proteins provide a biochemical indication of poor nutrition before the clinical signs are evident.I also look at the serum albumin, even though this is a relatively "long-lived" protein that takes longer to be affected by a nutritional deficit. It's part of my standard laboratory panel, however, so it's a readily available figure. It has been shown that low-serum albumin in hospitalized patients has been associated with longer hospital stays and sicker patients. A low-serum albumin not accounted for in other disease states, such as liver or kidney failure, is associated with a lowered immune response. Albumin is lowered in infections and often with cancer.

Results:

Retinol-binding protein	3.0-6.0 mg/dl
Transferrin	200-400 mg/dl

Albumin   3.5-5.0 gm/dl
                            (I like to see it
                            between 4.5 and
                            5.5 gm/dl.)

ImmunoMedex

The ImmunoMedex test is a special panel of blood tests that allows the physician to survey the inflammatory and nutritional response of the body and, therefore, predict the immune response.

Results:
    1 or less = very low risk
      2-10 = mild risk
    11-20 = medium risk
    21-30 = high risk
       30 = very high risk

Nutritional deficits, especially of protein, calories, vitamins and minerals, are frequently seen in hospitalized patients. These deficiencies adversely affect the immune system, lead to poor wound healing and coagulation problems, alter drug metabolism and increase the risk of disease and death. Nutritional shortcomings also decrease the patient's tolerance for chemotherapy and radiation, and they lengthen the convalescent time following surgery. Therefore, the ImmunoMedex test is an absolute must for most any ill person who is planning surgery or who wants an early indication of immune system weakness.

Immuno-Nutrition Measurements

I also look at what we call anthropometric measurements (measurements of the human body), which can be done in a doctor's office, or anywhere else for that matter. These simple measurements are used to estimate the nutritional status of a patient in terms of fat and protein reserves.

Height and Weight Measurements

We're all familiar with how height and weight are measured. Unfortunately, there is no specific formula for height and weight that will tell you if a person is obese or malnourished. Height and weight can only be used in a general way to estimate a person's status. Height-weight charts are flawed, but those of us in clinical medical nutrition need some sort of standard. The 1983 Metropolitan Life Insurance Reference Weights have been judged to be a satisfactory reference point.

Height (in inches)	Weight (in pounds)	
	Male	Female
58	-	114
59	-	116.5
60	-	119
61	-	122
62	133	125
63	135	128
64	137.5	131
65	140	134
66	143	137
67	146	140
68	149	143
69	152	146
70	155	149
71	158.5	152
72	162	-
73	166	-
74	169.5	-
75	174	-
76	179	-

Based on Reference Figures From the 1983
Metropolitan Height-Weight Tables

---

* Adapted from *Cecil Textbook of Medicine*, 17th ed, Ed. Wyngaarden, J., Smith, L. W. B. Saunders Co., Philadelphia, 1985, p. 1180.

Again, the height-weight tables are used only as a rough guide. The weight figures represent the middle of the range of weight for a medium built person of that height. Keep in mind that these figures were derived from men and women between the ages of 20 and 59 who purchased life insurance, and therefore they are not necessarily good guides for all ages and other groups.

As a general rule, weighing 20 percent more than the weight for your height suggests that you are obese. By this measure, roughly one in four Americans is obese. Weighing 20 percent less than the weight for your height groups suggests that you are underweight.

By this measure, roughly one in 20 Americans is underweight.

Triceps Skin Fat Thickness Test

Next is the triceps skin-fat thickness test, a method of estimating how many of the pounds a person weighs are accounted for by fat. In other words, what percentage of the body weight is fat as opposed to bone, muscle and so on. This is a very quick and easy test. The doctor or nurse uses a skin-fold caliper, which looks something like a pair of pliers with a meter attached. A bit of skin and fat on the arm at the triceps (the muscle on the back side of the upper arm) is pinched, the caliper is gently applied and a reading is taken. It takes only a moment, and it doesn't hurt at all. The goal is to measure the fat lying under the skin. Lean people will have little to pinch; hefty people will have more. Here are ideal figures:

Triceps Skinfold (in millimeters)*

	Ages 25-64	Ages over 65
Male	12	11
Female	21	24

* Summary of the finding of Frisancho, A.R. *Am. J. Clin. Nut.*, 34:2540, 1981.

Figures less than half those shown above support a diagnosis of malnourishment. Numbers twice or greater than those shown above support a diagnosis of obesity (and possibly overnourished/malnourished). In my office, I take skin-fold measurements from six different places on the body, and calculate the percentage of body fat from all six measurements.

Mid-Arm Muscle Circumference

The fourth anthropometric test to help ascertain nutritional status is measurement of mid-arm muscle circumference (MAMC), which estimates skeletal muscle mass. This is also a quick and easy test, in which a measuring tape is used to determine the circumference of the arm, midway between the elbow and the shoulder (where the triceps skin-fold measure was taken). Having measured the mid-arm circumference, the next step is to subtract the fat, which is represented by the triceps skin-fat thickness measurement. What remains represents muscle and lean body tissue. Plug your mid-arm circumference into this formula to derive your mid-arm muscle circumference:

$$\text{MAMC (cm)} = \frac{\text{mid-arm circumference}}{\text{(TSF [mm]} \times 0.314)}$$

MAMC = mid arm muscle circumference
TSF = triceps skin fold
cm = centimeter
mm = millimeters

Then take your MAMC and rate yourself on the chart below:

Mid-arm muscle circumference
(in centimeters)*

	Ages 25-64	Ages over 65
Male	27.9	26.8
Female	21.2	22.5

* Summary of the findings of Frisancho, A.R., *Am. J. Clin. Nut.*, 34:2540, 1981.

A MAMC of 20 percent or more below the numbers on the table above would help support a diagnosis of loss of lean body mass.

These four tests—height, weight, triceps skin fold and midarm circumference—are not the only anthropometric measurements that can be taken. But these four are quick and easy to do and provide a good starting point for further investigation.

What Do Deviations from the Norm Mean?

What does it mean when one or more of your laboratory tests is high or low? Any number of problems, organic, nutritional, stress-related, could be the cause. I wish I could give you a simple answer, but test results must be considered within the framework of a person's total medical evaluation. A complete personal and medical history, thorough physical examination and various other studies must be performed to make sure there is no organic reason for the deviation, and that the problem isn't stress-induced. Having ruled out an organic or stress-related disorder, I look for a nutritional explanation for the immune shortcomings.

You've Finished Reading the Book

The quest for lifelong, vibrant health and happiness is only beginning. I wish I could say that all you had to do was read Immune for Life and your troubles would vanish. Unfortunately, life doesn't work that way. Becoming immune for life requires your steadfast adherence to the program.

In the third section of this book you've learned a lot about the immune system. Integrate this information with what you've already discovered about the Immune for Life program and about yourself. The greater your understanding of the program, the easier it will be for you to stick with it.

Before you put this book down, please make a solemn promise to start taking care of yourself today. Make an unbreakable commitment to a lifetime of glowing health and happiness. Tell yourself that you deserve only the best in life, and that you're willing and eager to make yourself Immune for Life.

Bibliography

Nutrition, Vitamins and Minerals

Abramsky, O.: Common and uncommon neurological manifestations as presenting symptoms of vitamin B_{12} deficiency. *J. Am. Geriat. Soc.*, 20:93, 1972.

Ames, B. N.: Dietary carcinogens and anticarcinogens, oxygen radicals, and degenerative diseases. *Science*, 221:1256, 1983.

Anderson, C. F., Wochos, D. N.: The utility of serum albumin values in the nutritional assessment of hospitalized patients. *Mayo Clin. Proc.*, 57:181, 1982.

Anderson, J. A.: Nonimmunologically-mediated food sensitivity. *Nutr. Rev.*, 42:109, 1984.

Anderson, R.: Effects of ascorbate on leucocytes. II. Effects of ascorbic acid and calcium and sodium ascorbate on neutrophil phagocytosis and postphagocytosis and postphagocytic metabolic activity. *S. Afr. Med. J.*, 56:401, 1979.

Anderson, R.: Ascorbate-mediated stimulation of neutrophil motility and lymphocyte transformation by inhibition of the peroxidase/H_2O_2/halide system *in vitro* and *in vivo*. *Am. J. Clin. Nutr.*, 34:1906, 1981.

Anderson, R.: Effects of ascorbate on normal and abnormal leukocyte functions. *Int. J. Vitam. Nutr. Res.*, 23:23 (supp), 1982.

Anderson, R., Oosthuizen, R., Maritz, R., et al: The effects of increasing weekly doses of ascorbate on certain cellular and humoral immune functions in normal volunteers. *Am. J. Clin. Nutr.*, 33:71, 1980.

323

Anderson, R., Theron, A.: Effects of ascorbate on leucocytes. III. *In vitro* and *in vivo* stimulation of abnormal neutrophil motility by ascorbate. *S. Afr. Med. J.*, 56:429, 1979.

Anderson, R., Van Wyk, H.: The effects of ascorbate ingestion on levels of salivary IgA in adult volunteers. *(Letter) Am. J. Clin. Nutr.*, 33:6, 1980.

Anthony, L. E., Kurahara, C. G., Taylor, K. B.: Immunocompetence and ascorbic-acid deficiency in guinea pigs. *(Abstract) Fed. Proc.*, 37:931, 1978.

Antia, A., et al: Serum siderophilin in kwasiorkor. *Arch. Dis. Child.*, 43:459, 1968.

Axelrod, A. E.: The role of nutritional factors in the antibody responses of the anamnestic response. *Am. J. Clin. Nutr.*, 6:119, 1958.

Axelrod, A. E.: Immune processes in vitamin deficiency states. *Am. J. Clin. Nutr.*, 24:265, 1971.

Axelrod, A. E., Trakatellis, A. C., Block, H., et al: Effect of pyridoxine deficiency upon delayed hypersensitivity in guinea pigs. *J. Nutr.*, 79:161, 1963.

Ballester, D. E, Prasad, A. S.: Energy, zinc deficiency, and decreased nucleotide phosphorylase activity in patients with sickle-cell anemia. *Ann. Intern. Med.*, 98:180, 1983.

Banic, S., Kosak, M.: Prevention of transfusion hepatitis by vitamin C. *Int. J. Vit. Nutr. Res.*, 19:41 (supp) 1979.

Beach, R. S., et al: Growth and development of postnatally zinc-deprived mice. *Jour. Nutr.*, 110:201, 1980.

Beisel, W. R.: Magnitude of the host nutritional responses to infection. *Am. J. Clin. Nutr.*, 30:1236, 1977.

Beisel, W. R.: Single nutrients and immunity. *Am. J. Clin. Nutr.*, 35:417 (supp), 1982.

Beisel, W. R., Edelman, R., Nauss, K., et al: Single-nutrient effects on immunologic functions. *JAMA*, 245:53, 1981.

Bollag, W.: Effects of vitamin A acid on transplantable and chemically induced tumors. *Cancer Chemother. Rep.*, 55:53, 1971.

Bourry, J., Milano, G., Caldani, C., et al: Assessment of nutritional proteins during the parenteral nutrition of cancer patients. *Ann. Clin. Lab. Sci.*, 12:158, 1982.

Boxer, L. A., Vanderbilt, B., Bonsib, B., et al: Enhancement of chemotactic response and microtubule assembly in human leukocytes by ascorbic acid. *J. Cell. Physiol.*, 100:119, 1979.

Boxer, L. A., Watanabe, A. M., Bister, M., et al: Correction of leukocyte function in Chediak-Higashi syndrome by ascorbate. *New Engl. J. Med.*, 295:1041, 1976.

Brin, M.: Dilemma of marginal vitamin deficiency. *Proc. 9th Int. Congr. Nutr.*, 4:102, 1975.

Bristrain, B. R., Blackburn, G. L., Vitale, J., et al: Prevalence of malnutrition in general medical patients. *JAMA*, 235:1567, 1976.

Buckley, R. H.: Iron deficiency anemia: its relationship to infection susceptibility and host defense. *J. Pediatr.*, 86:993, 1975.

Campbell, P. A., Cooper, H. R., Heinzerling, R. H., et al: Vitamin E enhances *in vitro* immune response by normal and nonadherent spleen cells. *Proc. Soc. Exp. Biol. Med.*, 146:465, 1974.

Chandra, R. K.: Vitamin deficiencies. In Immunology of nutritional disorders, pp 55-106. Yearbook Pub., Chicago, 1980.

Chandra, R. K.: Lymphocyte subpopulations in malnutrition: cytotoxic and suppressor cells. *Pediatrics*, 59:423, 1977.

Chandra, R. K.: Immunodeficiency in undernutrition and overnutrition. *Nutr. Rev.*, 39:225, 1981.

Chandra, R. K.: Nutritional regulation of immunity and infection in the gastrointestinal tract. *J. Pediatr. Gastroenterol. Nutr.*, 2:181, 1983.

Chandra, R. K.: Nutritional regulation of immune function at the extremes of life: In infants and in the elderly. *In* Malnutrition: Determinants and Consequences, pp. 245-251, Alan R. Liss, New York, 1984.

Chandra, R. K., Au, B., Woodford, G., et al: Iron status, immunocompetence, and susceptibility to infection. *In* Iron Metabolism. Ciba Foundation Symposium, No. 51. Elsevier, Amsterdam, 1977.

Chandra, R. K., et al: Single nutrient deficiency and cell-mediated immune responses. II: Pyridoxine. *Nutr. Res.*, 1:101, 1981.

Chandra, R. K., Gupta, S., Singh, H.: Inducer and suppressor T-cell subsets in protein-energy malnutrition: analysis by monoclonal antibodies. *Nutr. Res.*, 2:21, 1982.

Chandra, R. K., Joshi, P., Au, B., et al: Nutrition and immunocompetence of the elderly. Effect of short-term nutritional supplementation on cell-mediated immunity and lymphocyte subsets. *Nutr. Res.*, 2:223, 1982.

Chandra, R. K., Kutty, K. N.: Immunocompetence in obesity. *Acta. Pediatr. Scand.*, 69:25, 1980.

Clemetson, C. A. B.: Histamine and ascorbic acid in the blood. *J. Nutr.*, 110:662, 1980.

Cohen, B. E., Cohen, I. K.: Vitamin A: Adjuvant and steroid antagonist in the immune response. *J. Immun.*, 111:1376, 1973.

Cohen, B. E., Elin, R. J.: Vitamin A-induced nonspecific resistance to infection. *J. Infect. Dis.*, 129:597, 1974.

Dionigi, R.: Immunological factors in nutritional assessment. *Proc. Nutr. Soc.*, 41:355, 1982.

Dresser, D. W.: Adjuvanticity of vitamin A. *Nature*, 217:527, 1968.

Douville, P., Talbot, J., Lapointe, R., et al: Potential usefulness of serum prealbumin in total parenteral nutrition. *Clin. Chem.*, 28:1706, 1982.

Dreblow, D. M., Anderson, C. E, Moxness, K.: Nutritional assessment of orthopedic patients. *Mayo Clin. Proc.*, 56:51, 1981.

Duchateau, J., Dilespesse, G., Vereeks, P.: Influence of oral zinc supplementation on the lymphocyte response to mitogens of normal subjects. *Am. J. Clin. Nutr.*, 34:88, 1981.

Edelman, R.: Cell mediated immune response in protein-calorie malnutrition: a review. In Malnutrition and the Immune Response, ed. Suskind, R. M., Raven Press, New York, 1975.

Fisher, M., Levine, P. H., Weiner, B., et al: The effect of vegetarian diets on plasma lipid and platelet levels. *Arch. Intern. Med.*, 146:1193, 1986.

Fox, A.: *The Beverly Hills Medical Diet.* Chain-Pinkham Books, St. Louis Park, Minnesota, 1981.

Fox, A.: The apple power team. How to win in life with nutrition and positive thinking. *Let's Live*, 5/82, p. 60.

Fox, A.: Vitamin C. *Let's Live*, 1/83, p. 36.

Fox, A.: Resistance to disease through nutrition. Part 1: Zinc. *Let's Live*, 10/83, p. 23.

Fox, A.: Resistance to disease through nutrition. Part 2: Phenylalanine. *Let's Live*, 11/83, p. 16.

Fox, A.: Resistance to disease through nutrition. Part 3: Copper. *Let's Live*, 12/83, p. 10.

Fox, A.: Resistance to disease through nutrition. Part 4: Beta carotene. *Let's Live*, 1/84, p. 20.

Fox, A.: Resistance to disease through nutrition. Part 5: The B complex. *Let's Live*, 2/84, p. 18.

Fox, A.: Resistance to disease through nutrition. Part 6: Magnesium. *Let's Live*, 3/84, p. 47.

Fox, A Resistance to disease through nutrition. Part 7: Selenium. *Let's Live*, 4/84, p. 32.

Fox, A.: Resistance to disease through nutrition. Part 8: Your calcium bank. *Let's Live*, 5/84, p. 34.

Fraser, R. C., Pavlovic, S., Kurahara, C. G., et al: The effect of variations in vitamin C intake on the cellular immune response of guinea pigs. *Am. J. Clin. Nutr.*, 33:839, 1978.

Golden, M. H. N., Golden, B. E.: Zinc and immunocompetence in protein-energy malnutrition. Lancet, 1:1226, 1978.

Jain, V. K., Chandra, R. K.: Hypothesis: Does nutritional deficiency predispose to acquired immune deficiency syndrome? *Nutr. Res.*, 4:537, 1984.

Kay, N., et al: Endorphins stimulate normal human peripheral blood lymphocyte. *Life Science*, 35(1):53, 1984.

Knapp, H. R., Reilly, I. A., Alessandrini, P.: *In vivo* indexes of platelet and vascular function during fish-oil administration in patients with atherosclerosis. *New Engl. J. Med.*, 314:937, 1986.

Kromhout, D., Bosschieter, E.B., et al: The inverse relationship between fish consumption and 20-year mortality from coronary heart disease. *New Engl. J. Med.*, 312:1205, 1985.

Lytle, L. D., Altar, A.: Diet, central nervous system, and aging. *Fed. Proc.*, 38:2017, 1979.

McCoy, J. H., Kenney, M. A.: Depressed immune response in magnesium-deficient rats. *Jour. Clin. Nutr.*, 105:791, 1975.

Merritt, R. J., et al: Consequences of modified fasting in obese pediatric and adolescent patients. Effect of a carbohydrate-free diet on serum proteins. *Am. J. Clin. Nutr.*, 34:2752, 1981.

Mulhern, S. A., et al: Influence of selenium and chow diets on immune function in first and second generation mice. *Fed. Proc., Fed. Am. Soc. Exp. Biol.,* 40:935, 1981.

Prasad, J. S.: Effect of vitamin E supplementation on leukocyte function. *Am. J. Clin. Nutr.,* 33:606, 1980.

Rosenberg, I. H., Solomons, N. W., Schneider, R.: Malabsorption associated with diarrhea and intestinal infections. *Am. J. Clin. Nutr.,* 30:1248, 1977.

Sirisinha, S.: Immunoglobluins and complement in protein-calorie malnutrition. *In* Protein-calorie malnutrition, pp. 369-375, Academic Press, New York, 1975.

Sheffy, B. E., Schultz, R. D.: Influence of vitamin E and selenium on immune response mechanisms. *Fed. Proc.,* 38:2139, 1979.

Shekelle, R. B., Missell, L., et al: Fish consumption and mortality from coronary heart disease. *New Engl. J. Med.,* 313:820, 1985.

Smith, R. E, Suskina, R., Thanagkul, O., et al: Plasma vitamin A., retinol-binding protein and prealbumin concentrations in protein-calorie malnutrition, III: Response to varying dietary treatmerits. *Am. J. Clin. Nutr.,* 28:732, 1975.

Waterlow, J. C., Alleyne, G. A. O.: Protein malnutrition in children: Advances in knowledge in the last ten years. *Adv. Protein. Chem.,* 25:117, 1971.

Watson, R. R., Leonard, T. K.: Vitamin A, E and C: nutrients with cancer prevention properties. *J. Am. Diet. Assoc.,* 86:505, 1986.

Watson, R. R., Moriguchi, S.: Cancer prevention by retinoids: role of immunological modification. *Nutr. Res.,* 5:663, 1985.

Weinsier, R. L., Hunker, E. M., Krundieck, C. L., et al: Hospital malnutrition: a prospective evaluation of general medical patients during the course of hospitalization. *Am. J. Clin. Nutr.,* 32:418, 1979.

Whitehead, R. G., Alleyne, G. A. O.: Pathophysiological factors of importance in protein-calorie malnutrition. *Brit. Med. Bull.,* 28:72, 1972.

Willard, M. D., Gilsdorf, R. B., Price, R. A.: Protein-calorie malnutrition in a community hospital. *JAMA,* 243:1720, 1980.

Woods, H. E: Biochemical methods in nutritional assessment. *Proc. Nutr. Soc.,* 41:419. 1982.

Worthington, B. S.: Effect of nutritional status on immune phenomena. *J. Am. Dietet. Assn.,* 65:123, 1974.

Immune System

Anderson, R.: Effects of ascorbate on leucocytes. II. Effects of ascorbic acid and calcium and sodium ascorbate on neutrophil phagocytosis and post-phagocytosis and post-phagocytic metabolic activity. *S. Afr. Med. J.,* 56:401, 1979.

Anderson, R.: Ascorbate-mediated stimulation of neutrophil motility and lymphocyte transformation by inhibition of the peroxidase/H_2O_2/ halide system *in vitro* and *in vivo. Am. J. Clin. Nutr.,* 34:1906, 1981.

Anderson, R.: Effects of ascorbate on normal and abnormal leukocyte functions. Int. J. Vitam. *Nutr. Res.,* 23:23 (supp), 1982.

Anderson, R., Oosthuizen, R., Maritz, R., et al: The effects of increasing weekly doses of ascorbate on certain cellular and humoral immune functions in normal volunteers. *Am. J. Clin. Nutr.*, 33:71, 1980.

Anderson, R., Theron, A.: Effects of ascorbate on leucocytes. Ill. *In vitro* and *in vivo* stimulation of abormal neutrophil motility by ascorbate. *S. Afr. Med. J.*, 56:429, 1979.

Anderson, R., Van Wyk, H.: The effects of ascorbate ingestion on levels of salivary IgA in adult volunteers. (Letter) *Am. J. Clin. Nutr.*, 33:6, 1980.

Anthony, L. E., Kurahara, C. G., Taylor, K. B.: Immunocompetence and ascorbic-acid deficiency in guinea pigs. (Abstract) *Fed. Proc.*, 37:931, 1978.

Axelrod, A. E.: The role of nutritional factors in the antibody responses of the anamnestic response. *Am. J. Clin. Nutr.*, 6:119, 1958.

Axelrod, A. E.: Immune processes in vitamin deficiency states. *Am. J. Clin. Nutr.*, 24:265, 1971.

Axelrod, A. E., Trakatellis, A. C., Block, H., et al: Effect of pyridoxine deficiency upon delayed hypersensitivity in guinea pigs. J. Nutr., 79:161, 1963.

Ballester, D. E, Prasad, A. S.: Energy, zinc deficiency, and decreased nucleotide phosphorylase activity in patients with sickle-cell anemia. *Ann. Intern. Med.*, 98:180, 1983.

Barnes, D. M.: Nervous and immune-system disorders linked in a variety of diseases. *Science*, 232:160, 1986.

Beisel, W. R.: Magnitude of the host nutritional responses to infection. *Am. J. Clin. Nutr.*, 30:1236, 1977.

Beisel, W. R.: Single nutrients and immunity. *Am. J. Clin. Nutr.*, 35:417 (supp), 1982.

Beisel, W. R., Edelman, R., Nauss, K., et al: Single-nutrient effects on immunologic functions. *JAMA*, 245:53, 1981.

Boxer, L. A., Vanderbilt, B., Bonsib, B., et al: Enhancement of chemotactic response and microtubule assembly in human leukocytes by ascorbic acid. *J. Cell. Physiol.*, 100:119, 1979.

Boxer, L. A., Watanabe, A. M., Bister, M., et al: Correction of leukocyte function in Chediak-Higashi syndrome by ascorbate. *New Engl. J. Med.*, 295:1041, 1976.

Buckley, R. H.: Iron deficiency anemia. Its relationship to infection susceptibility and host defense. *J. Pediatr.*, 86:993, 1975.

Campbell, P. A., Cooper, H. R., Heinzerling, R. H., et al: Vitamin E enhances *in vitro* immune response by normal and nonadherent spleen cells. *Proc. Soc. Exp. Biol. Med.*, 146:465, 1974.

Chandra, R. K.: Immunocompetence in undernutrition. *J. Pediatr.*, 8:1194, 1972.

Chandra, R. K.: Rosette forming T-lymphocytes and cell-mediated immunity in malnutrition. *Br. Med. J.*, 3:608, 1974.

Chandra, R. K.: Lymphocyte subpopulations in malnutrition: cytotoxic and suppressor cells. *Pediatrics*, 59:423, 1977.

Chandra, R. K.: Immunodeficiency in undernutrition and overnutrition. *Nutr. Rev.* 39:225, 1981.

Chandra, R. K.: Nutritional regulation of immunity and infection in the gastrointestinal tract. *J. Pediatr. Gastroenterol. Nutr.*, 2:181, 1983.

Chandra, R. K.: Nutritional regulation of immune function at the extremes of life: In infants and in the elderly. *In* Malnutrition: Determinants and Consequences, pp. 245-251, Alan R. Liss, New York, 1984.

Chandra, R. K., Au, B., Woodford, G., et al: Iron status, immunocompetence, and susceptibility to infection. *In* Iron Metabolism. Ciba Foundation Symposium, No. 51. Elsevier, Amsterdam, 1977.

Chandra, R. K., et al: Single nutrient deficiency and cell-mediated immune responses. II: Pyridoxine. *Nutr. Res.*, 1:101, 1981.

Chandra, R. K., Gupta, S., Singh, H.: Inducer and suppressor T cell subsets in protein-energy malnutrition: analysis by monoclonal antibodies. *Nutr. Res.*, 2:21, 1982.

Chandra, R. K., Joshi, P., Au, B., et al: Nutrition and immunocompetence of the elderly. Effect of short-term nutritional supplementation on cell-mediated immunity and lymphocyte subsets. *Nutr. Res.*, 2:223, 1982.

Chandra, R. K., Kutty, K. N.: Immunocompetence in obesity. *Acta. Paediatr. Scand.*, 69:25, 1980.

Clemetson, C. A. B.: Histamine and ascorbic acid in the blood. *J. Nutr.*, 110:662, 1980.

Cohen, B. E., Cohen, 1. K.: Vitamin A: Adjuvant and steroid antagonist in the immune response. *J. Immun.*, 111:1376, 1973.

Cohen, B. E., Elin, R. J.: Vitamin A-induced nonspecific resistance to infection. *J. Infect. Dis.*, 129:597, 1974.

Dionigi, R.: Immunological factors in nutritional assessment. *Proc. Nutr. Soc.*, 41:355, 1982.

Duchateau, J., Dilespesse, G., Vereeks, P.: Influence of oral zinc supplementation on the lymphocyte response to mitogens of normal subjects. *Am. J. Clin. Nutr.*, 34:88, 1981.

Doull, J., Klaassen, C. D., Amdur, M. O., eds.: *Casarett and Doull's Toxicology*, 2nd ed. Macmillan Publishing Co., New York, 1980.

Edelman, R.: Cell mediated immune response in protein-calorie malnutrition: a review. *In* Malnutrition and the Immune Response, ed. Suskind, R. M., Raven Press, New York, 1975.

Fauci, A. S., Macher, A. M., Longo, D. L., et al: Acquired immuno-deficiency syndrome: Epidemiologic, clinical, immunologic, and therapeutic considerations. *Intern. Med.*, 100:92, 1984.

Fraser, R. C., Pavlovic, S., Kurahara, C. G., et al: The effect of variations in vitamin C intake on the cellular immune response of guinea pigs. *Am. J. Clin. Nutr.*, 33:839, 1978.

Golden, M. H. N., Golden, B. E.: Zinc and immunocompetence in protein-energy malnutrition. *Lancet*, 1:1226, 1978.

Jain, V. K., Chandra, R. K.: Hypothesis: Does nutritional deficiency predispose to acquired immune deficiency syndrome? *Nutr. Res.*, 4:537, 1984.

Johansson, S. G. O.: Immunological mechanisms of food sensitivity. *Nutr. Rev.*, 42:79, 1984.

Marx, J. L.: The Immune System "Belongs in the Body." *Science*, 227:1190, 1985.

McCoy, J. H., Kenney, M.A.: Depressed immune response in magnesium. deficient rats. *Jour. Clin. Nutr.*, 105:791, 1975.

Miller, G. C.: Enkephalins-enhancement of active T-cell rosettes from normal volunteers. *Clin. Immun.-Immunopath.*, 31:132, 1984.

Miller, J. A.: Immunity and crises, large and small. *Science News*, 129:340, 1986.

Mulhern, S. A., et al: Influence of selenium and chow diets on immune function in first and second-generation mice. *Fed. Proc., Fed. Am. Soc. Exp. Biol.*, 40:935, 1981.

Pessimistic attitude toward adversity may predispose to poor immune function, illness, early mortality. *Int. Med. News*, 19:10, 1986.

Plotnikoff, N. P., et al: Enkephalins: immunomodulators. *Fed. Proc.*, 44 (1 pt. 1):118, 1985.

Prasad, J. S.: Effect of vitamin E supplementation on leukocyte function. *Am. J. Clin. Nutr.*, 33:606, 1980.

Ruff, M. R., et al: Opiate receptor-mediated chemotaxis of human monocytes. *Neuropeptides*, 5:363, 1985.

Sheffy, B. E., Schultz, R. D.: Influence of vitamin E and selenium on immune response mechanisms. *Fed. Proc.*, 38:2139, 1979.

Simkins, C. O., et al: Human neutrophil migration is enhanced by betaendorphin. *Life Science*, 34:2251, 1984.

Sirisinha, S.: Immunoglobluins and complement in protein-calorie malnutrition. *In* Protein-calorie malnutrition, pp. 369-375, Academic Press, New York, 1975.

Smith, R. E, Suskina, R., Thanagkul, O., et al: Plasma vitamin A, retinol-binding protein and prealbumin concentrations in protein-calorie malnutrition, III: Response to varying dietary treatments. *Am. J. Clin. Nutr.*, 28:732, 1975.

Waddell, C. C., et al: Inhibition of lymphoproliferation by hyperlipoprotienemia plasma. *Jour. Clin. Invest.*, 58:950, 1976.

Walford, R. L.: Immunologic theory of aging: current status. *Fed. Proc., Fed. Am. Soc. Exp. Biol.*, 33:2020, 1974.

Worthington, B. S.: Effect of nutritional status on immune phenomena. *J. Am. Dietet. Assn.*, 65:123, 1974.

Disease

Ames, B. N.: Dietary carcinogens and anticarcinogens, oxygen radicals, and degenerative diseases. *Science*, 221:1256, 1983.

Bailar, J. C, Smith, E. M.: Progress against cancer? *New Engl. J. Med.*, 314:1226, 1986.

Baker, R. W., Peppercorn, M. A.: Gastrointestinal ailments of homosexual men. *Medicine*, 61:390, 1982.

Banic, S., Kosak, M.: Prevention of transfusion hepatitis by vitamin C. Int. J. Vit. Nutr. Res., 19:41 (supp), 1979.

Bernard, D. Z. J., Leibowitch, J., Safai, B., et al: HTLV-III in cells cultured from semen of two patients with AIDS. *Science*, 226:449, 1984.

Boxer, L. A., Watanabe, A.M., Bister, M., et al: Correction of leukocyte function in Chediak-Higashi syndrome by ascorbate. *New Engl. J. Med.*, 295:1041, 1976.

Center For Disease Control: Kaposi's sarcoma and Pneumocystis pneumonia among homosexual men New York and California. *Morbid Mortal. Weekly Rep.*, 30:305, 1981.

Dritz, S. K., Goldsmith, R. S.: Sexually transmissible protozoal, bacterial, and viral enteric infections. *Compr. Ther.*, 6:34, 1980.

Fox, A., Fox, B.: The high cost of disease: prevention is cheaper than a by-pass. *Let's Live*, 3/86, p. 10.

Groopman, J. E.: Causation of AIDS revealed. *Nature*, 308:769, 1984.

Harris, C., Small, C. B., Klein, R. S., et al: Immunodeficiency in female sexual partners of men with the acquired immunodeficiency Syndrome. *New Engl. J. Med.*, 308:1181, 1984.

Hill, G. L., Pickford, I., Young, G.A., et al: Malnutrition in surgical patients: an unrecognized problem. *Lancet*, 1:689, 1977.

Hoskins, L. C., Winawer, S. J., Broitman, S. A., et al: Clinical giardiasis and intestinal malabsorption. *Gastroenterology*, 53:265, 1967.

Jain, V. K., Chandra, R. K.: Hypothesis: Does nutritional deficiency predispose to acquired immune deficiency syndrome? *Nutr. Res.*, 4:537, 1984.

Knapp, H. R., Reilly, I. A., Alessandrini, P.: *In vivo* indexes of platelet and vascular function during fish-oil administration in patients with atherosclerosis. *New Engl. J. Med.*, 314:937, 1986.

Kromhout, D., Bosschieter, E. B., et al: The inverse relationship between fish consumption and 20-year mortality from coronary heart disease. *New Engl. J. Med.*, 312:1205, 1985.

Lopez, C., Fitzgerald, P. A., Siegal, E P.: Severe acquired immune deficiency syndrome in male homosexuals: Diminished capacity to make interferon-alpha *in vitro* associated with severe opportunistic infections. *J. Infect. Dis.*, 48:962, 1983.

Lyon, J. L., Klauber, M. R., Gardner, J. W., et al: Cancer incidence in Mormons and non-Mormons in Utah. *New Engl. J. Med.*, 294:129, 1976.

Rosenberg, I. H., Solomons, N. W., Schneider, R.: Malabsorption associated with diarrhea and intestinal infections. *Am. J. Clin. Nutr.*, 30:1248, 1977.

Rubinstein, A., Sicklick, M., Gupta, A., et al: Acquired immuno-deficiency with reversed T4/T8 ratios in infants born to promiscuous and drug-addicted mothers. *JAMA*, 249:2350, 1983.

Shekelle, R. B., Missell, L., et al: Fish consumption and mortality from coronary heart disease. *New Engl. J. Med.*, 313:820, 1985.

Watson, R. R., Leonard, T. K.: Vitamin A, E and C: nutrients with cancer prevention properties. *J. Am. Diet. Assoc.*, 86:505, 1986.

Watson, R. R., Moriguchi, S.: Cancer prevention by retinoids: role of immunological modification. *Nutr. Res.*, 5:663, 1985.

Weinsier, R. L., Hunker, E. M., Krundieck, C. L., et al: Hospital malnutrition: a prospective evaluation of general medical patients during the course of hospitalization. *Am. J. Clin. Nutr.*, 32:418, 1979.

Whitehead, P.. G., Alleyne, G. A. O.: Pathophysiological factors of importance in protein-calorie malnutrition. *Brit. Med. Bull.*, 28:72, 1972.

Willard, M. D., Gilsdorf, R. B., Price, R. A.: Protein-calorie malnutrition in a community hospital. *JAMA*, 243:1720, 1980.

Endorphins and DLPA

Fox, A., Fox, B.: Endorphins and pain. *Let's Live*, 12/84, p. 24.

Fox, A., Fox, B.: *DLPA to End Chronic Pain and Depression*. Long Shadow Books, New York, 1985.

Fox, A., Fox, B.: Natural relief for pain and depression—phenylalanine. *Let's Live*, 1/85, p. 10.

Fox, A., Fox, B.: The latest on DLPA. *Let's Live*, 12/85, p. 34.

Kay, N., et al: Endorphins stimulate normal human peripheral blood lymphocyte. *Life Science*, 35(1):53, 1984.

Miller, G. C.: Enkephalins-enhancement of active T-cell rosettes from normal volunteers. *Clin. Immun.-Immunopath.*, 31:132, 1984.

Plotnikoff, N. P., et al: Enkephalins: immunomodulators. *Fed. Proc.*, 44(1 pt. 1):118, 1985.

Ruff, M. R., et al: Opiate receptor-mediated chemotaxis of human monocytes. *Neuropeptides*, 5:363, 1985.

Simkins, C. O., et al: Human neutrophil migration is enhanced by beta-endorphin. *Life Science*, 34:2251, 1984.

Wybran, J.: Enkephalins and endorphins: activation molecules for the immune system and natural killer activity. *Neuropeptides*, 5:371, 1985.

The Mind

Barnes, D. M.: Nervous and immune system disorders linked in a variety of diseases. *Science*, 232:160, 1986.

Fox, A.: The apple power team. How to win in life with nutrition and positive thinking. *Let's Live*, 5/82, p. 60.

Fox, A.: The Biochemical Proof for Positive Thinking. *Creative Thought*, 62(1):8, 1985.

Fox, A., Fox, B.: Endorphins and pain. *Let's Live*, 12/84, p. 24.

Fox, A., Fox, B.: *Wake Up! You're Alive*. Health Communications, Florida, 1988.

Level of burn recovery linked to attitude of patient. *Am. Med. News*, May 9, 1986, p. 48.

Miller, J. A.: Immunity and crises, large and small. *Science News*, 129:340, 1986.

Pessimistic attitude toward adversity may predispose to poor immune function, illness, early mortality. *Int. Med., News* 19:10, 1986.

Index

Index of Recipes